# PROVISION OF MENTAL HEALTH COUNSELING SERVICES UNDER TRICARE



Committee on the Qualifications of Professionals Providing Mental Health Counseling Services Under TRICARE

Board on the Health of Select Populations

INSTITUTE OF MEDICINE
*OF THE NATIONAL ACADEMIES*

THE NATIONAL ACADEMIES PRESS
Washington, D.C.
**www.nap.edu**

**THE NATIONAL ACADEMIES PRESS 500 Fifth Street, N.W. Washington, DC 20001**

NOTICE: The project that is the subject of this report was approved by the Governing Board of the National Research Council, whose members are drawn from the councils of the National Academy of Sciences, the National Academy of Engineering, and the Institute of Medicine. The members of the committee responsible for the report were chosen for their special competences and with regard for appropriate balance.

This study was supported by a contract between the National Academy of Sciences and the US Department of Defense via HHS award HHSP23320080006T, TO#24. Any opinions, findings, conclusions, or recommendations expressed in this publication are those of the authors and do not necessarily reflect the view of the organizations or agencies that provided support for this project.

International Standard Book Number-13: 978-0-309-14766-8
International Standard Book Number-10: 0-309-14766-2

Additional copies of this report are available from the National Academies Press, 500 Fifth Street, NW, Lockbox 285, Washington, DC 20055; (800) 624-6242 or (202) 334-3313 (in the Washington metropolitan area); Internet, http://www.nap.edu.

For more information about the Institute of Medicine, visit the IOM home page at: **www.iom.edu.**



Printed in the United States of America

*Cover credit:* Image © Neville Elder/Corbis.

The serpent has been a symbol of long life, healing, and knowledge among almost all cultures and religions since the beginning of recorded history. The serpent adopted as a logotype by the Institute of Medicine is a relief carving from ancient Greece, now held by the Staatliche Museen in Berlin.

Suggested citation: IOM (Institute of Medicine). 2010. *Provision of Mental Health Counseling Services Under TRICARE.* Washington, DC: The National Academies Press.

*"Knowing is not enough; we must apply.*
*Willing is not enough; we must do."*
—Goethe

INSTITUTE OF MEDICINE
*OF THE NATIONAL ACADEMIES*

**Advising the Nation. Improving Health.**

# THE NATIONAL ACADEMIES

***Advisers to the Nation on Science, Engineering, and Medicine***

The **National Academy of Sciences** is a private, nonprofit, self-perpetuating society of distinguished scholars engaged in scientific and engineering research, dedicated to the furtherance of science and technology and to their use for the general welfare. Upon the authority of the charter granted to it by the Congress in 1863, the Academy has a mandate that requires it to advise the federal government on scientific and technical matters. Dr. Ralph J. Cicerone is president of the National Academy of Sciences.

The **National Academy of Engineering** was established in 1964, under the charter of the National Academy of Sciences, as a parallel organization of outstanding engineers. It is autonomous in its administration and in the selection of its members, sharing with the National Academy of Sciences the responsibility for advising the federal government. The National Academy of Engineering also sponsors engineering programs aimed at meeting national needs, encourages education and research, and recognizes the superior achievements of engineers. Dr. Charles M. Vest is president of the National Academy of Engineering.

The **Institute of Medicine** was established in 1970 by the National Academy of Sciences to secure the services of eminent members of appropriate professions in the examination of policy matters pertaining to the health of the public. The Institute acts under the responsibility given to the National Academy of Sciences by its congressional charter to be an adviser to the federal government and, upon its own initiative, to identify issues of medical care, research, and education. Dr. Harvey V. Fineberg is president of the Institute of Medicine.

The **National Research Council** was organized by the National Academy of Sciences in 1916 to associate the broad community of science and technology with the Academy's purposes of furthering knowledge and advising the federal government. Functioning in accordance with general policies determined by the Academy, the Council has become the principal operating agency of both the National Academy of Sciences and the National Academy of Engineering in providing services to the government, the public, and the scientific and engineering communities. The Council is administered jointly by both Academies and the Institute of Medicine. Dr. Ralph J. Cicerone and Dr. Charles M. Vest are chair and vice chair, respectively, of the National Research Council.

**www.national-academies.org**

## COMMITTEE ON THE QUALIFICATIONS OF PROFESSIONALS PROVIDING MENTAL HEALTH COUNSELING SERVICES UNDER TRICARE

**GEORGE J. ISHAM** (*Chair*), Medical Director and Chief Health Officer, Health Partners, Inc., Bloomington, Minnesota

**KATHRYN K. BASHAM,** Professor, Smith College School of Social Work, Northampton, Massachusetts

**ALISA B. BUSCH,** Assistant Professor of Psychiatry and of Health Care Policy, Harvard Medical School and McLean Hospital; Director of Integration of Clinical Measurement and Health Services Research, McLean Hospital, Belmont, Massachusetts

**N. EMMANUEL G. CASSIMATIS,** President and CEO, Educational Commission for Foreign Medical Graduates, Philadelphia, Pennsylvania

**JOHN H. MOXLEY III,** Independent Consultant, Solvang, California

**HAROLD A. PINCUS,** Professor and Vice Chair, Department of Psychiatry and Associate Director, Irving Institute for Clinical and Translational Research, Columbia University; Director of Quality and Outcomes Research, New York Presbyterian Hospital, New York, New York

**THEODORE P. REMLEY, JR.,** Professor and Batten Endowed Chair in Counseling, Department of Educational Leadership and Counseling, Old Dominion University, Norfolk, Virginia

**PHYLLIS W. SHARPS,** Professor and Chair, Department of Community Public Health Nursing, Johns Hopkins University School of Nursing, Baltimore, Maryland

**ROY A. SWIFT,** Senior Director, Personnel Credentialing Accreditation Programs, American National Standards Institute, Washington, DC

**VILIA M. TARVYDAS,** Professor, Counseling, Rehabilitation, and Student Development, College of Education, University of Iowa, Iowa City, Iowa

***Consultant***

**RHONDA J. ROBINSON BEALE,** Chief Medical Officer, OptumHealth Behavioral Solutions, Glendale, California

*Program Staff*

**DAVID A. BUTLER,** Senior Program Officer; Study Director
**JESSICA L. BUONO,** Research Associate (until August 2009)
**SARAH GAILLOT,** Christine Mirzayan Science and Technology Policy Fellow
**ANDREW BRADLEY,** Intern
**TIA S. CARTER,** Senior Program Assistant
**PAMELA RAMEY-McCRAY,** Administrative Assistant
**FREDERICK (RICK) ERDTMANN,** Director, Board on the Health of Select Populations and Medical Follow-up Agency
**NORMAN GROSSBLATT,** Senior Editor

# Reviewers

This report has been reviewed in draft form by persons chosen for their diverse perspectives and technical expertise in accordance with procedures approved by the National Research Council's Report Review Committee. The purpose of the independent review is to provide candid and critical comments that will assist the institution in making its published report as sound as possible and to ensure that the report meets institutional standards of objectivity, evidence, and responsiveness to the study charge. The review comments and draft manuscript remain confidential to protect the integrity of the deliberative process. We thank the following for their review of the report:

**Paula G. Allen-Meares,** Chancellor, University of Illinois at Chicago
**Dwight L. Evans,** Chairman, Department of Psychiatry, University of Pennsylvania School of Medicine
**Samuel Templeman (Sam) Gladding,** Professor and Chair of Counseling, Wake Forest University
**Sharon M. Goldsmith,** President, Goldsmith International SP
**Michael A. Hoge,** Professor of Psychology and Director, Yale Behavioral Health, Yale University
**Kevin C. Kiley,** Associate Professor and Chairman of the Department of Obstetrics and Gynecology, Albany Medical College

**Janice L. Krupnick,** Professor of Psychiatry and Director, Trauma and Loss Program, Georgetown University

**Richard A. McCormick,** Consultant, Clinical Psychologist, and Senior Scholar, Center for Health Care Research and Policy, Case Western Reserve University

**Robert J. Ursano,** Chair, Department of Psychiatry, Uniformed Services University of the Health Sciences

**Myrna M. Weissman,** Professor of Epidemiology and Psychiatry, Columbia University College of Physicians and Surgeons, and Chief, Department of Clinical-Genetic Epidemiology, New York State Psychiatric Institute

**Reg Arthur Williams,** Professor of Acute, Critical and Long Term Care Programs, School of Nursing and Professor of Psychiatry, Medical School, University of Michigan

Although the reviewers listed above have provided many constructive comments and suggestions, they were not asked to endorse the conclusions or recommendations, nor did they see the final draft of the report before its release. The review of the report was overseen by **Dan G. Blazer,** J.P. Gibbons Professor of Psychiatry, Duke University Medical Center, and **Paul S. Appelbaum,** Elizabeth K. Dollard Professor of Psychiatry, Medicine, and Law, Columbia University. Appointed by the National Research Council and the Institute of Medicine, they were responsible for making certain that an independent examination of the report was carried out in accordance with institutional procedures and that all review comments were carefully considered. Responsibility for the final content of the report rests with the authoring committee and the institution.

# Acknowledgments

This report could not have been prepared without the guidance and expertise of numerous persons. Although it is not possible to mention by name all those who contributed to the committee's work, the committee wants to express its gratitude to a number of them for their special contributions.

Sincere thanks go to all the participants at the public meetings convened on April 9 and July 7, 2009. The intent of the workshops was to gather information regarding issues related to the practice of mental health counselors in various care setting. The speakers, who are listed in Appendix A, gave generously of their time and expertise to help inform and guide the committee's work. Many of them also provided additional information in response to the committee's myriad questions.

We are indebted to Rhonda Robinson-Beale, who served as a consultant to the committee and who shared her deep knowledge of the provision of mental health–care services in managed-care settings.

The committee extends special thanks to the dedicated and hardworking staff of the Institute of Medicine's Board on the Health of Select Populations, who supported and facilitated its work. Board Director Rick Erdtmann helped to ensure that this report met the highest standards of quality.

Finally, the committee members would like to thank the chair, George Isham, for his outstanding work, leadership, and dedication to this project.

# Contents

## APPENDIXES

# Summary

The physical and mental rigors associated with military service take their toll on the men and women who defend the country, the families that support them, and those who have retired from active duty. The responsibility for providing health care to that population rests with TRICARE. TRICARE is an integrated, single-payer health-services provider that combines the health-care resources of military treatment facilities with networks of civilian health-care professionals, medical facilities, and suppliers.

TRICARE's beneficiary population is large and diverse. As of 2009, it encompassed some 9.5 million people in the United States and abroad. Only about 20% are active-duty members of the armed forces or activated members of the National Guard or Reserves; the remainder are family members of those groups (26%) and retirees and their families (54%). Almost half are female. The population spans a range of ages: 21% are under 18 years old, and 20% are over 64 years old.

The mental health–care needs of that population are equally large and diverse. Warfighters are vulnerable to a variety of complex and sometimes difficult-to-diagnosis conditions, including posttraumatic stress disorder and traumatic brain injury. Stresses resulting from multiple and long deployments put military families at risk for marital conflict, intimate-partner violence, and behavioral disturbances in children. Age-related changes in health and personal circumstances open retirees to depression.

Those needs are met by a set of professionals who have different education, training, and expertise. Among them are mental health counselors, who—like clinical social workers, marriage and family therapists, and psychiatric nurse specialists—typically hold master's degrees and are obligated by state licensure and other requirements to have demonstrated clinical experience in order to practice. They provide services to individuals and groups through psychotherapy,[1] behavior modification, and other systematic intervention strategies.

Federal code and TRICARE policy require counselors[2] to deliver services subject to a physician's referral and supervision for them to be eligible for reimbursement. That distinguishes counselors from some other providers.

## INTENT AND GOALS OF THE STUDY

In 2008, Congress directed the Department of Defense (DOD) to ask the Institute of Medicine (IOM) to conduct a study of the credentials, preparation, and training of people who were practicing as licensed mental health counselors and to make recommendations for permitting these counselors to practice independently under the TRICARE program. In response, IOM formed and convened the Committee on the Qualifications of Professionals Providing Mental Health Counseling Services Under TRICARE.

In TRICARE, independent practice frees providers from requirements that state that a beneficiary must be "referred for therapy by a physician" and that the referring physician "must actually see the patient to evaluate and diagnose the condition to be treated prior to referring the beneficiary" and provide "ongoing oversight of the course of referral related treatment throughout the period during which the beneficiary is being treated," including "ongoing communication between the

---

[1]This report uses the term *psychotherapy* interchangeably with *counseling*, following the convention applied by most of the literature. Some sources differentiate between the two, however, and definitions are provided where needed.

[2]This report uses the term *counselors* to identify persons who are more formally referred to as *mental health counselors* or *professional counselors*. The education, training, licensing, and certification requirements for counselors are addressed in Chapter 3. This chapter also differentiates the requirements for counselors from those applied to other mental health professionals.

referring and treating provider" (32 CFR § 199.6). TRICARE recognizes psychiatrists and other physicians, clinical psychologists, certified psychiatric nurse specialists, clinical social workers, and certified marriage and family therapists working under a participation agreement as independent providers of mental health services.

DOD provided the committee with a statement of task that requested assessments of the educational, licensing, and clinical-experience requirements imposed on mental health counselors and the extent to which they are authorized to practice independently under other federal health-care programs. The statement of task also asked for a review of the history of regulations under which mental health–care providers are recognized under TRICARE, data on the percentage of patients under the care of counselors, and a review of studies of the comparative outcomes and effectiveness of care provided by counselors. Finally, it requested that the committee offer conclusions and recommendations for permitting counselors to practice independently under TRICARE, including any limitations on that practice. DOD did not ask for an analysis of and the committee did not address issues surrounding access to mental health care.

## REPORT SYNOPSIS

### Mental Health Issues in the TRICARE Beneficiary Population

The committee's statement of task identified a set of illnesses for attention in assessing the education, licensure, and clinical experience of and the quality and effectiveness of care provided by counselors:

- Major depressive disorder;
- Schizophrenia;
- Posttraumatic stress disorder;
- Bipolar disorder;
- Mental disorders due to a general medical condition;
- Somatoform disorders; and
- Delirium, dementia, amnestic, substance-use, and other disorders regularly associated with head trauma.

Those illnesses may be caused or exacerbated by physical and psychological exposures related to military service. They present challenges for all health professionals. Their diagnosis may be difficult because of overlapping symptoms between multiple distinct mental health disorders or between mental and general health disorders. Treatment in some cases entails pharmacologic and other medical interventions—which are outside the ambit of counselors, marriage and family therapists, clinical social workers, and, in some circumstances, other nonphysician practitioners—rather than or in addition to psychological care. For such conditions as bipolar disorder or schizophrenia, for example, evidence-based practice recommends that patients receive medication to minimize symptoms or prevent repeated episodes of illness. For other conditions—such as major depression, substance-use disorders, and anxiety disorders—medications can be efficacious, but patients with symptoms or exacerbations may also be adequately treated with psychosocial interventions alone. Often, patients can benefit from a combination of medications and psychosocial treatment. The committee noted that evidence-based psychosocial interventions exist for schizophrenia and for major depressive, acute stress, posttraumatic stress, bipolar, substance-use, generalized anxiety, obsessive-compulsive, and panic disorders.

The committee's research also found other disorders that TRICARE beneficiaries are at special risk for. These psychosocial problems—which include issues related to interpersonal relationships, behavior, and stress—fall more directly in counseling's primary focus on promoting coping and facilitating growth related to life-cycle transitions.

The diversity and the diagnostic and treatment complexity of the mental health illnesses found in the beneficiary population highlight the need for a comprehensive approach to quality management in care delivery in the TRICARE system.

### Education, Licensing, and Clinical-Experience Requirements

The statement of task requested the committee to perform assessments of the educational, licensure, and clinical-experience requirements imposed on counselors. Those requirements are essential components of a credentialing system that helps to establish whether a professional is prepared to practice. They are also components of a system of quality management for a care provider.

The field of counseling comprises several specialties in educational and career guidance and clinical care. Educational requirements for graduate programs in mental health counseling vary by institution. Admission requirements include a bachelor's degree and some combination of a minimum grade-point average and standardized test scores, successful completion of relevant preparatory coursework, letters of recommendation, personal interviews, and evidence of interest in the field as demonstrated by volunteer work and the like. Graduation requirements typically mirror a state's requirements to apply for entry-level licensure as a mental health counselor. They include successful completion of core curricula and a minimum number of course, practicum, and related training and experience hours.

Some graduate programs in mental health counseling are accredited by the Council for Accreditation of Counseling and Related Educational Programs (CACREP), an independent agency created by the profession. The educational requirements and curricula for mental health counselors who graduated from institutions that are CACREP-accredited in mental health counseling or clinical mental health counseling (after July 1, 2009) contain elements relevant to preparing counselors to serve as independent practitioners and to diagnose and treat for disorders that may be found in the TRICARE beneficiary population. These include knowledge—and the skills and practices needed to implement knowledge—of

- The etiology, diagnostic process and nomenclature, treatment, referral, and prevention of mental and emotional disorders.
- The principles of the diagnostic process, including differential diagnosis, and the use of current diagnostic tools, such as the current edition of the *Diagnostic and Statistical Manual of Mental Disorders* (*DSM*).
- Evidence-based treatments and basic strategies for evaluating counseling outcomes in clinical mental health counseling (CACREP, 2009).

Licensure requirements for mental health counselors vary by state. In general, they comprise

- A master's degree or higher degree in mental health counseling or sometimes a related field.
- A minimum number of semester hours of coursework—either 48 or 60.

- Adherence to a state or national organization's code of ethics or conduct.
- A number of hours of supervised and total professional experience.
- Passage of one or more examinations of professional competence.

Some states require a minimum number of hours of patient contact or continuing education per year for license renewal. There are considerable differences among the states in the details of the requirements. Typically, only those in higher or the highest licensure level for a state may diagnose and treat patients independently. Codes of ethics or conduct and in some cases state laws require counselors to provide services only within their competencies and scope of practice, to diagnose properly, to educate themselves in and apply scientifically based treatment modalities, and to appropriately refer patients who present with problems outside their competencies and scope of practice.

Two examinations are commonly used to assess fitness for licensure. The more rigorous, the National Clinical Mental Health Counselor Examination (NCMHCE), comprises clinical simulations that span the diverse characteristics of the TRICARE beneficiary population. The NCMHCE requires experience and competencies that are desirable in persons who serve as independent practitioners and diagnose and treat for mental and substance-use (M/SU) disorders that may be found in the TRICARE beneficiary population.

TRICARE's clinical-experience requirements for licensed counselors comprise "two years of post-masters experience which includes 3000 hours of clinical work and 100 hours of face-to-face supervision" [32 CFR § 199.6(c)(3)(iv)(C)(*2*)]. The requirements mirror those specified for a person holding certification as a Certified Clinical Mental Health Counselor, a voluntary credential administered by a professional organization of counselors, and they are similar to those imposed by states for the higher or highest level of licensure as a mental health counselor.

The research reviewed by the committee indicates that—although education, licensing, and clinical-experience requirements play roles in a system of quality management—there is no information that would allow one to determine whether a particular education level, licensure, or amount of clinical experience is needed to serve effectively as an independent practitioner or to establish whether a practitioner is adequately prepared to diagnose and treat disorders that may be found in the TRICARE beneficiary population. In general, the training of the mental health practitioners varies, and fulfillment of education, licensure, and clinical-experience requirements does not ensure exposure to particular disorders or competence in treating for them.

### Independent and Supervised Practice of Counselors in Other Health-Care Systems

The statement of task asked the committee to assess the extent to which counselors practice independently in other settings and to review the history of the regulation of mental health–care providers by TRICARE.

Programs such as Medicare, those administered by the Department of Veterans Affairs, the Indian Health Service, and Head Start, and those provided under the Federal Employee Health Benefits Program and by private insurers exhibit no consistent pattern in their policies regarding the independent practice of counselors. The policies are by and large driven by federal, state, and tribal laws and regulations and by institutional practice. In the case of private insurers, recognition of members of particular professions as independent practitioners for the purpose of billing is sometimes determined by the organization that contracts for coverage.

A historical review of the regulations prescribed by DOD regarding the recognition of mental health providers as independent practitioners indicates that policy is driven primarily by congressional mandate. In the one circumstance in which members of a nondoctoral-level mental health profession (clinical social workers) were granted independent-practice authority by both TRICARE and Medicare, the profession was granted authority under TRICARE before Medicare. Congress directed that the authority be granted in both circumstances.

No conclusions relevant to the topic of the independent practice of counselors under TRICARE can be drawn from the experience of other federal programs or of private insurers.

### Clinical Exposure and Capability Studies

The committee could not identify any published data regarding the number or proportion of patients who had particular mental health disorders that were under the care of counselors. TRICARE provided some data in response to a request from the committee, which are presented in Table 2.16. As the text accompanying the table notes, the data are of limited usefulness. Generally, the committee believes that such information would not answer the question of whether or under what circumstances counselors should be permitted to provide independent services under TRICARE inasmuch as it does not address the quality of care or the ability of counselors to provide high-quality care.

The committee sought to identify outcome studies and literature regarding the comparative quality and effectiveness of care provided by licensed mental health counselors. It found that a number of meta-analyses and reviews had examined psychotherapy and counseling effectiveness, but they do not provide evidence on the comparative effectiveness of treatment by different types of mental health–care providers. Arguments of differential effectiveness by mental health–care provider type are generally not based on empirical evidence but are instead based on anecdotal information or supposition. Research suggests that experience may have a favorable effect on diagnostic accuracy, but it has consistently demonstrated that the variance observed in treatment outcomes is primarily the result of variance in the effectiveness of individual therapists.

## Research Regarding Quality of Care

Available information indicates that supervision of counselors under TRICARE's current requirements is "highly varied" and that "compliance with the supervision requirement [is] more of a formality than a valuable exercise" (Meredith et al., 2005). A 2006 DOD report to Congress indicated that physician oversight of counselors' clinical work "occurs predominantly on paper" and "is difficult to ensure to any great degree" (DOD, 2006). The analyses suggest that supervision requirements neither affect quality of care nor add to the protection of beneficiaries.

An earlier IOM report (2006) indicated that there are serious deficiencies in the health and behavioral health infrastructure that affect quality of care. It found that the education of all health professionals was lacking. The report specifically noted that "not all M/SU clinicians are educated about evidence-based care or receive training in the use of evidence-based clinical practice guidelines" and "quality improvement strategies have received little attention in M/SU education." It identified a need for an infrastructure to collect and disseminate the new knowledge and clinical information required to deliver high-quality patient care and to facilitate quality-measurement and quality-improvement activities.

DOD's Mental Health Task Force also identified problems in the military's system of care, finding that "the TRICARE network benefit for psychological health is hindered by fragmented rules and policies" and that "there are not sufficient mechanisms in place to assure the use of evidence-based treatments or the monitoring of treatment effectiveness" (DOD, 2007).

Care providers, including the Military Health System (MHS), use delineated scopes of practice and privileging of individual practitioners to ensure that all health professionals deliver the services that they have demonstrated competence in. Previous IOM reports in the *Quality Chasm* series indicate that the best way for health-care providers like TRICARE to achieve the delivery of high-quality care to their beneficiaries is through appropriate standards of education and training for providers, promotion of evidence-based care standards, and monitoring of results (IOM, 2001, 2006).

## Overall Conclusions and Recommendations

Education, accreditation, licensure, certification, and clinical-experience requirements for mental health professionals are components of a quality-management system. However, they have little specificity with regard to knowledge of and experience with particular health problems or evidence-based practices. That generally limits the confidence that can be placed in the preparation of *any* of these professionals to diagnose and treat disorders that may be found in the TRICARE beneficiary population. Research regarding the quality of care for M/SU conditions indicates that there are widespread deficiencies in the training of providers and in the infrastructure that supports their practice.

The committee did not identify any evidence that distinguishes mental health counselors from other classes of practitioners in ability to serve in an independent professional capacity or to provide high-quality care consistent with education, licensure, and clinical experience. Its research instead points to the need for a comprehensive quality-management system that facilitates the proper diagnosis of and treatment for disorders in the TRICARE beneficiary population by all mental health practitioners.

The committee was tasked to offer

> conclusions and recommendations for permitting licensed mental health counselors to practice independently under the TRICARE program, including recommendations regarding modifications of current policy for the TRICARE program with respect to allowing licensed mental health counselors to practice independently in the TRICARE program, paying particular attention to the preparedness of licensed mental health counselors to diagnose, treat, and appropriately refer persons with disorders of particular importance to TRICARE beneficiaries.

In light of the information that it gathered and reviewed, it recommends that TRICARE replace its current quality management system for oversight of the practice of counselors through physician referral and supervision with a mental health quality monitoring and management system that incorporates the following two primary elements:

**[1] Independent practice of mental health counselors in TRICARE in the circumstances in which their education, licensure, and clinical experience have helped to prepare them to diagnose and, where appropriate, treat conditions in the beneficiary population.** Those circumstances comprise

- A master's or higher-level degree in counseling from a program in mental health counseling or clinical mental health counseling that is accredited by CACREP.
- A state license in mental health counseling at the "clinical" or the higher or highest level available in states that have tiered licensing schemes.
- Passage of the NCMHCE.
- A well-defined scope of practice for practitioners.

The scope of practice should be based on a systematic assessment of the professional and cultural competencies necessary to address the mental and behavioral health needs of the TRICARE beneficiary population and should include the types of patients that can be seen, the settings in which they can be seen, and the interventions and populations (including pediatric, adolescent, and geriatric) that the practitioner has demonstrated competency in.

The committee believes that it is important to maintain continuity of care for TRICARE beneficiaries who are receiving services from counselors under the current system. It therefore recommends that TRICARE institute a strategy that allows for the continuing service of practitioners who did not graduate from CACREP-accredited programs,[3] have not attained "clinical" or similar licensure, or have not successfully completed the NCMHCE. TRICARE may, for example, wish to conduct supervision of such professionals by using a model patterned after Army Regulation 40–68, Sections 7–6c and d (Appendix E), which provides for successively greater levels of independent practice as experience and demonstrated competence increase.

**[2] A comprehensive quality-management system for all mental health professionals.** This system should include

- Well-defined scopes of practice and clinical privileging of all mental health–care providers in the direct and purchased-care systems that are consistent with professional education, training, and experience, where these scopes are not already present.
- Promotion of evidence-based practices for treatment of conditions and monitoring of results.
- Focused training in the particular mental and related general medical conditions that are present in the TRICARE beneficiary population and in military cultural competence.
- A systematic process for continued professional education and training to ensure continuing improvement in the clinical evidence base and accommodation of the changing needs of the TRICARE population.
- Development and application of quality measures to assess the performance of providers.

---

[3]Some current counselors may have graduated from programs accredited by the Council on Rehabilitation Education, later gained clinical experience and earned licensure in mental health counseling, and be practicing as counselors. The committee does not intend to exclude such persons from practicing in the TRICARE system.

- Systematic monitoring of the process and outcomes of care at all levels of the health-care system and application of effective quality-improvement strategies.

The committee notes that the recommendations regarding evidence-based practices, training and education, quality measures, and monitoring echo the observations offered by the DOD Task Force on Mental Health (DOD, 2007). DOD publications and public pronouncements (Casscells, 2008; DOD, 2008) indicate that MHS is already pursuing these recommendations as part of its efforts to implement best practices in quality management. For example, the DOD Center for Deployment Psychology (CDP) is currently offering courses on military cultural competence to TRICARE personnel and other MHS practitioners (CDP, 2009). In April 2010, CDP will initiate a military and veteran behavioral health post-master's certificate program that will "teach best clinical practices to mental health professionals who are addressing the behavioral health needs of military personnel, veterans and their families" and include training in military culture, combat trauma, suicidal risk, and blast-related traumatic brain injury (TBI) (CDP, 2010). The committee believes that the framework necessary to support the independent practice of counselors under the circumstances delineated above is thus already being put into place, that TRICARE should be able to implement the recommended policy changes in a timely manner, and that it should do so because of the critical mental health needs in its beneficiary population. As a step toward achieving the comprehensive system recommended here, the TRICARE Management Activity should consider requiring that organizations demonstrate that they have mechanisms in place to promote the delivery of evidence-based care, to apply quality measures to assess the performance of providers, to monitor outcomes, and to implement improvement strategies as a condition of their provider contracts.

The committee observes that the barriers to establishing a robust quality infrastructure for mental health care are common to all providers and suggests that TRICARE may benefit from working with other government organizations—such as the Department of Veterans Affairs and the Department of Health and Human Services' Agency for Healthcare Research and Quality, Centers for Medicare and Medicaid Services, National Institutes of Health, and Substance Abuse and Mental Health

Services Administration—to conduct or support research to overcome the barriers.

## REFERENCES

CACREP (Council for Accreditation of Counseling and Related Educational Programs). 2009. *CACREP accreditation manual. 2009 standards.* Alexandria, VA: Council for Accreditation of Counseling and Related Educational Programs.

Casscells SW. 2008. *Statement on mental health by the Honorable S. Ward Casscells, MD. Assistant Secretary of Defense for Health Affairs, before the Subcommittee on Military Personnel of the Armed Services Committee, U.S. House of Representatives,* March 14. http://www.dod.mil/dodgc/olc/docs/testCasscells080314.pdf. (Accessed October 9, 2009).

CDP (Center for Deployment Psychology, Department of Defense). 2009. *Welcome to the Center for Deployment Psychology.* http://www.deploymentpsych.org/. (Accessed 22 December 2009).

CDP. 2010. *Military and veteran behavioral health post-master's certificate program.* http://postgraduatecenter.org/MVBH%20Certificate.html. (Accessed January 15, 2010).

DOD (Department of Defense). 2006. *Aspects of the use of licensed professional counselors in the Military Health System. Report to Congress.* Transmittal letter, August 28. http://www.tricare.mil/planning/congress/downloads/2006/new/Licensed-Mental.pdf. (Accessed October 20, 2009).

DOD. 2007. *An achievable vision: Report of the Department of Defense Task Force on Mental Health.* Falls Church, VA: Defense Health Board. www.health.mil/dhb/mhtf/MHTF-Report-Final.pdf. (Accessed October 27, 2009).

DOD. 2008. *The Military Health System strategic plan. A roadmap for medical transformation.* http://www.health.mil/StrategicPlan/2008%20Strat%20Plan%20Final%20-lowres.pdf. (Accessed October 27, 2009).

IOM (Institute of Medicine). 2001. *Crossing the quality chasm: A new health system for the 21st century.* Washington, DC: National Academy Press.

IOM. 2006. *Improving the quality of health care for mental and substance-use conditions: Quality chasm series.* Washington, DC: The National Academies Press.

Meredith LS, Tanielian T, Greenberg MD, Suarez A, Eiseman E. 2005. *Expanding access to mental health counselors: Evaluation of the TRICARE demonstration.* Santa Monica, CA: RAND Corporation.

# 1

# Introduction

This chapter addresses the provision of mental health care services under TRICARE, the military's medical services delivery system. It begins with an overview of the TRICARE program and then provides basic information on TRICARE's mental health services and the professionals that provide them, with a focus on governing statutes and regulations. The statement of task for the Institute of Medicine (IOM) committee responsible for this report is presented next, followed by the committee's approach to responding to it. The chapter concludes with brief summaries of related IOM reports and a description of the present report's organization. Many of the topics touched on in this chapter are addressed in greater detail in later chapters.

## TRICARE'S RESPONSIBILITIES AND STRUCTURE[1]

TRICARE is the US Department of Defense (DOD) health-care benefits program for all seven uniformed services—the Army, the Navy, the Marine Corps, the Air Force, the Coast Guard, the Commissioned Corps of the Public Health Service, and the Commissioned Corps of the

[1]General information in this section is derived from the *TRICARE Beneficiary Handbook* (TRICARE, 2009b) and other materials on the TRICARE Web site: http://www.tricare.mil. This chapter contains a brief summary of the information as it existed when the report was written; TRICARE sources should always be consulted for authoritative materials.

National Oceanic and Atmospheric Administration—and the National Guard and Reserves. It is the contemporary embodiment of a commitment to provide care for the country's defense and fighting force that extends back to 1775 and has evolved to extend services to the larger military family (DOD, 2009). TRICARE had its origins in demonstration projects and a reform initiative implemented in the 1980s in the Civilian Health and Medical Program of the Uniformed Services (CHAMPUS).[2] Its integrated system grew out of what had been disparate programs that provided care to active-duty personnel via military health facilities and to their dependents, retirees,[3] and other eligible persons via a network of military and civilian providers. The program's services combine the health-care resources of military treatment facilities (MTFs)—referred to as the direct-care component—with networks of civilian health-care professionals, medical facilities, and suppliers—the purchased-care component.

TRICARE operates as a single-payer system and covers most inpatient and outpatient medical care that is deemed necessary by a medical professional, including emergency and urgent care, medical and surgical procedures received on an inpatient basis and an outpatient basis, home health care, hospice care, clinical preventive services, maternity care, pharmacy services, and behavioral health care services (TRICARE, 2009b). The TRICARE program is managed by the TRICARE Management Activity (TMA) under the DOD assistant secretary of defense for health affairs. It is organized into six geographic health-service regions. The three regions in the United States are TRICARE North, TRICARE South, and TRICARE West; and the regions abroad are TRICARE Europe, TRICARE Latin America and Canada, and TRICARE Pacific. Each region is responsible for overseeing the administration and management of TRICARE health services, funding regional initiatives to improve the delivery of health-care services,

---

[2]CHAMPUS is still referred to in some regulatory and policy documents that address TRICARE operations.

[3]The US Office of Personnel Management offers the following somewhat circular definition of a military retiree: "any member or former member of the uniformed services who is entitled, under statute, to retired, retirement, or retainer pay on account of service as a member, or who receives military retired or retainer pay" (OPM, 2009). Eligibility for retiree status is usually determined by length of service (typically, 20 years or more), although there are other circumstances in which a service member may qualify. Military retirees are a subset of military veterans.

and supporting the operations of MTFs and civilian health-care centers that deliver care to beneficiaries in their regions.

In each region, a single provider is responsible for delivering purchased-care services under contract to the program. As of the middle of 2009, Health Net Federal Services managed health-care services for about 3.0 million beneficiaries in the north region, Humana Military Healthcare Services for 2.9 million in the south region, and TriWest Healthcare Alliance for 2.7 million in the west region (*Stars and Stripes,* 2009). In July 2009, it was announced that new contracts had been awarded to Aetna Government Health Plans for the north region, UnitedHealth Military & Veterans Services for the south region, and TriWest for the west region.

To access coverage, people must have their eligibility status recorded in the Defense Enrollment Eligibility Reporting System (DEERS) and have valid uniformed-services identification cards that display their eligibility. The two main categories of beneficiaries are sponsors and family members. Sponsors—who are active-duty service members, National Guard or Reserve members, or retirees—are automatically registered in DEERS; their dependents are not. Sponsors are responsible for ensuring that eligible family members are registered in DEERS for them to receive coverage.

Four separate programs under TRICARE provide different options for health-care services, addressing both the diverse needs of the beneficiary population and participants' preferences as to level and form of coverage. Coverage for active-duty service members, their families, and retirees under 65 years old is provided by TRICARE Prime, a managed-care option in which MTFs are the principal source of health care; TRICARE Extra, a preferred-provider option; and TRICARE Standard, a fee-for-service option. TRICARE for Life provides supplementary health-care coverage for TRICARE beneficiaries 65 years old and older who are entitled to Medicare Part A and enrolled in Medicare Part B; it offers full coverage for many services only partially covered by Medicare. All active-duty, National Guard, and Reserve service members are automatically enrolled in TRICARE Prime. Military dependents and retirees under 65 years old have the option of choosing from TRICARE Prime, TRICARE Extra, and TRICARE Standard. Table 1.1 lists eligible beneficiaries, available coverage options, and restrictions, if any, on benefits under the TRICARE program.

TRICARE policies regarding providers, covered persons, and procedures are defined by statute as set forth in the *United States Code* (USC),

**TABLE 1.1** Health-Care Coverage Under TRICARE

| Eligible Beneficiary | Coverage Options |
|---|---|
| Active-duty service member | TRICARE Prime |
| Active-duty family member (includes spouses, unmarried children up to 21 years old or 23 years old if enrolled in college full-time)<br>Uniformed-services retiree under 65 years old, eligible family members | TRICARE Prime<br>TRICARE Extra<br>TRICARE Standard |
| Dependent parent, parent-in-law | TRICARE Plus[a] |
| Active-duty service member who lives and works more than 50 miles or 1 hour's drive from a military treatment facility | TRICARE Prime Remote |
| Family member who resides with an active-duty service member who lives and works more than 50 miles or 1 hour's drive from a military treatment facility | TRICARE Prime Remote for Active Duty Service Members (TPR ADSM)<br>TRICARE Extra<br>TRICARE Standard |
| Active-duty member of the Reserves | TRICARE Prime<br>TRICARE Prime Remote |
| Family of a Reserve member activated for more than 30 days | TRICARE Prime<br>TPRADSM<br>TRICARE Extra<br>TRICARE Standard |
| Retired National Guard or Reserve member, family[b] | TRICARE Prime<br>TRICARE Extra<br>TRICARE Standard<br>TRICARE For Life (TFL) if 65 years old or older |
| Medicare-eligible beneficiary under 65 years old | TRICARE Prime<br>TRICARE Extra<br>TRICARE Standard |
| Medicare-eligible beneficiary 65 years old or older | TFL |
| Congressional Medal of Honor recipient, immediate family<br>Unremarried former spouse of active or retired military-service member | TRICARE Prime<br>TRICARE Extra<br>TRICARE Standard<br>TFL (if 65 years old or older) |
| Family of court-martialed sponsor | Eligibility determined case by case |
| Family of sponsor missing in action | Eligibility determined case by case |

**TABLE 1.1** Continued

| Eligible Beneficiary | Coverage Options |
|---|---|
| Foreign force member, family[c] | Coverage, eligibility depend on country of origin |
| Survivor | Benefits differ depending on survivor status entered in DEERS |
| Victim of abuse[d] | Eligible for limited medical benefits |

[a]TRICARE Plus is available only at certain military treatment facilities and allows beneficiaries who normally are able to get care at a military treatment facility only on a space-available basis to enroll and receive primary-care appointments with the same access standards as beneficiaries enrolled in TRICARE Prime.
[b]A sponsor and family members are not eligible for TRICARE health benefits until the sponsor reaches the age of 60 years and begins to receive retired pay.
[c]Must be registered in DEERS and have a valid military ID card.
[d]Care may be provided if the victim's active-duty spouse has been separated from the service for an abuse-related offense. The care must be related to an injury or illness caused by the abuse.
SOURCE: TRICARE (2009b). Note that several versions of the *TRICARE Beneficiary Handbook* are extant, addressing different regions and specific programs. An online version of this information is also available: http://www.tricare.mil/mybenefit/.

by regulations specified in the *Code of Federal Regulations* (CFR), and by instructions contained in TMA documents, such as the TRICARE operations, policy, reimbursement, and systems manuals.[4] Specific policies regarding behavioral health care are discussed in greater detail in the following section and chapters.

## MENTAL HEALTH–CARE SERVICES AND PROVIDERS UNDER TRICARE

A number of mental health services are covered under TRICARE; most of them are subject to limitations regarding the time, duration, or number of sessions covered per episode, admission, benefit period, or fiscal year (TRICARE, 2009a). Outpatient services include psychotherapy (individual, group, family, and conjoint therapy and collateral visits),

[4]Online versions of the manuals are maintained at http://manuals.tricare.osd.mil/.

psychoanalysis, psychological testing, and medication management. Inpatient services incorporate acute care, psychiatric partial hospitalization, and residential treatment-center care. In addition, a number of substance-use services are covered: inpatient detoxification and rehabilitation; outpatient care; individual, group, and family therapy; and psychiatric partial hospitalization. Coverage limitations are in many cases defined by statute; specifics are in Title 10 of the USC and Title 32 of the CFR.

Authorized providers recognized under TRICARE are defined in 32 CFR Part 199 and, generally, the *TRICARE Policy Manual* 6010.54-M, Chapter 11, Section 1.1. For mental health services, they comprise psychiatrists and other physicians, clinical psychologists, certified psychiatric nurse specialists, clinical social workers, certified marriage and family therapists, pastoral counselors, and mental health counselors (32 CFR § 199.4(c)(3)(ix) and *TRICARE Policy Manual* 6010.54-M, Chapter 7,

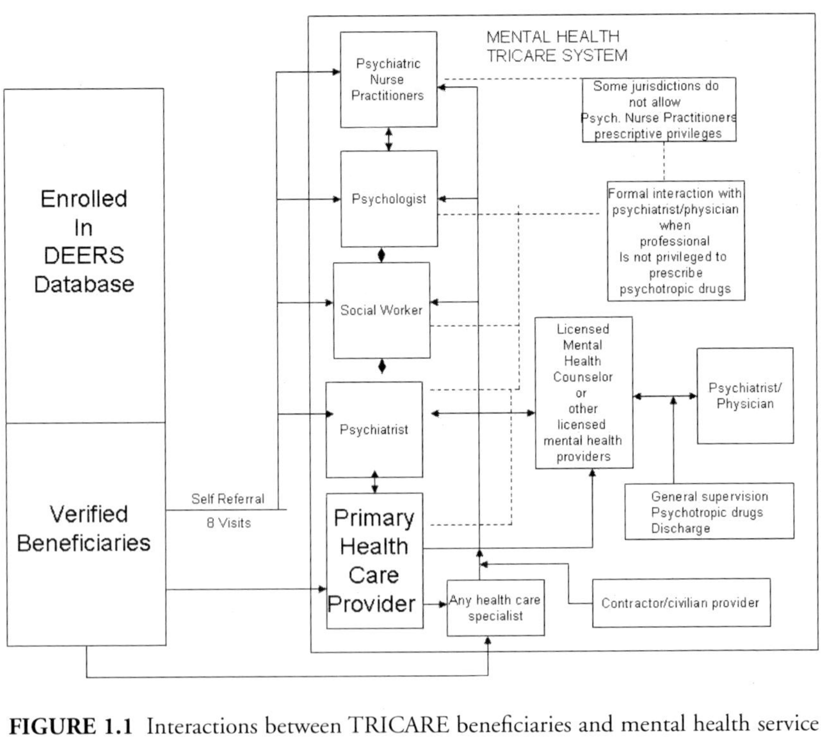


**FIGURE 1.1** Interactions between TRICARE beneficiaries and mental health service providers.

Section 3.10). Figure 1.1 schematically illustrates the interaction between beneficiaries and those professionals. Table 1.2 outlines the restrictions on their practice under TRICARE. Specific information on the scope of practice and training, experience, and licensing requirements for each type of provider is delineated below. Appendix D contains excerpts from 32 CFR § 199.6 that detail these requirements. Additional detail on the education of mental health professionals is provided in Chapter 3.

## Psychiatrists and Other Physicians

Psychiatrists are certified in the prevention, diagnosis, and treatment of mental, addictive, and emotional disorders and are qualified to assess both the physical and mental aspects of mental illness. They are differentiated from other mental health professionals by their medical training and can prescribe medications, perform physical examinations, and order laboratory tests and imaging studies. Training includes education that leads to a medical or osteopathic degree from an accredited university and at least 4 years in a psychiatric residency program (AADPRT, 2009). Authorization under TRICARE requires a medical or osteopathic degree, completion of an approved psychiatric residency program, and licensure by the state in which the person practices (*TRICARE Policy Manual* 6010.54-M, Chapter 11, Addendum A(2)(B), 2002). Psychiatrists and other physicians may apply for board certification in psychiatry or a subspecialty of their choosing, but it is not required.

As noted in the section on primary-care providers (PCPs) below, physicians trained or board-certified in other specialties may also be involved in mental health care and making diagnoses and in some cases may deliver treatment.

Title 32 of the CFR requires that "clinicians providing individual, group, and family therapy meet CHAMPUS requirements as qualified mental health providers and operate within the scope of their licenses." It goes on to state (32 CFR § 199.6(b)(4)(vii)(B)(*1*)(*i*)) that

> [t]he ultimate authority for planning, development, implementation, and monitoring of all clinical activities is vested in a psychiatrist or doctoral level psychologist. The management of medical care is vested in a physician.

**TABLE 1.2** Mental Health Professionals Under TRICARE—Disciplines and Associated Restrictions

| Discipline[a] | Requires Supervision and Referral by Physician | Need Participation Agreement to Practice Independently | Able to Supervise Applicable Staff |
|---|---|---|---|
| Licensed physician (including psychiatrist) | — | No | Yes |
| Licensed clinical psychologist | No | No | Yes |
| Licensed/certified psychiatric nurse specialists | No | No | Yes |
| Licensed/certified clinical social worker | No | No | Yes |
| Licensed/certified marriage and family therapist | No if participation agreement is signed; yes if participation agreement is not signed | Yes | Yes if participation agreement is signed; no if participation agreement is not signed |
| Licensed/certified pastoral counselor | Yes | No | Yes[b] |
| Licensed/certified mental health counselor | Yes | No | Yes |

[a]Licensure/certification must be at full clinical level of practice.
[b]If supervisee is not able to work toward licensure with discipline of supervisor, supervisor cannot supervise under TRICARE standards; supervisor must also be working within scope of his or her practice/license/certification.
SOURCE: NQMC (2005).

## Psychologists

Clinical psychologists perform many of the same functions as psychiatrists in developing treatments and interventions for people with mental health problems. However, they focus mainly on counseling, psychotherapy, rehabilitation, and behavior modification, and they are generally not permitted to prescribe medications (except those licensed and practicing in Louisiana, New Mexico, and Guam).[5] They also interpret psychological tests, such as intelligence examinations, personality tests, and brain-function assessments.

Clinical psychologists must have a doctoral degree (PhD or PsyD) in psychology or a closely related field. Graduate training includes practicum courses that provide clinical experience in counseling and diagnostic testing and an internship that involves working directly with clients under the supervision of a licensed psychologist. Clinical psychologists are able to obtain licensure after completing the required training and passing a state licensing examination (APA, 2009; BLS, 2008-09a). To be certified under TRICARE, clinical psychologists must be licensed or certified in psychology by the state in which they practice and have 2 years of supervised clinical experience in psychological health services, or they must be credentialed by the National Registry of Health Service Providers in Psychology (*TRICARE Policy Manual* 6010.54-M, Chapter 11, Section 3.7, 2002). These providers are able to deliver services under TRICARE without physician supervision.

## Psychiatric Nurse Specialists

Psychiatric nurse specialists provide advanced treatment for mental health disorders or behavioral health problems through psychotherapy and management of medications. They may perform direct inpatient care and couple, family, and group therapy, and they may serve as consultants, evaluators, and resources for staff nurses. Some have prescription privileges. Psychiatric nurse specialists are prepared as PCPs in psychiatric settings. The American Nurses Credentialing Center offers certification in adult psychiatric and mental health and in family psychiatric and mental health to nurse practitioners; clinical nurse

---

[5]In addition, the DOD Psychopharmacology Demonstration Project, which took place in 1991–1997, graduated 10 students from its pharmacotherapy training program and granted them privileges (Ralph and Sammons, 2006).

specialists may be certified in adult psychiatric and mental health and in child/adolescent psychiatric and mental health.

Under TRICARE, they are able to provide covered care without physician referral and supervision. Authorization requires licensure as a registered nurse (RN) and a master's degree (MS, MSN, or MN) or doctoral degree (PhD) in nursing with a specialization in psychiatric and mental health nursing. Additional training requirements include 2 years of post–master's degree experience with an average of 8 hours of direct patient contact per week (*TRICARE Policy Manual* 6010.54-M, Chapter 11, Section 3.6, 2002). They must also be certified by the American Nurses Association through the American Nurses Credentialing Center, which requires a minimum of 500 clinical hours in psychiatric and mental health nursing under faculty supervision during the graduate program; coursework in advanced health assessment, advanced pharmacology, and advanced pathophysiology; and clinical training in at least two psychotherapeutic treatment modalities . To practice psychotherapy, certification and 800 hours of direct patient contact in advanced clinical practice are required (American Nurses Credentialing Center, 2009).

## Clinical Social Workers

Clinical social workers, also referred to as mental health and substance-abuse social workers, provide diagnosis, biopsychosocial assessment, and treatment for people with mental illness and substance-abuse problems through individual, couple, family, and group therapy and rehabilitation. Practitioners must have a master's degree (MSW, MSSA, or MSS) from an accredited program that includes coursework in clinical assessment, counseling, psychotherapy, and caseload management. Additional training typically includes a minimum of 900 hours of supervised clinical field experience (BLS, 2008-09b). To be authorized under TRICARE, certification or licensure at the master's level is required by the state in which the provider practices. Licensing requirements vary by state; however, most require at least 2 years or 3,000 hours of post–master's degree clinical social-work practice under the supervision of a master's-level social worker in a clinical setting, which satisfies TRICARE requirements (*TRICARE Policy Manual* 6010.54-M, Chapter 11, Section 3.5, 2002). Clinical social workers authorized under TRICARE are able to provide covered care within the scope of their licenses without physician referral and supervision.

A note accompanying the requirements directs that "patients' organic medical problems must receive appropriate concurrent management by a physician."

**Marriage and Family Therapists**

Marriage and family therapy is recognized by the federal government as a "core" mental health profession, as are psychiatry, psychology, social work, and psychiatric nursing (HHS, 2009). Marriage and family therapists are trained in psychotherapy and family systems. They may assess, diagnose, and treat mental and emotional disorders through brief, solution-focused, family-centered treatment but are not authorized to prescribe medications (American Association for Marriage and Family Therapy, 2009). To become a marriage and family therapist, a person must earn a master's or doctoral degree in counseling with a focus on marriage and family therapy from a graduate program accredited by the Commission on Accreditation for Marriage and Family Therapy Education.

Licensure or certification requires 2 years of post–master's degree supervised clinical experience. Training requirements include a combination of 200 hours of approved supervision and 1,000 hours of supervised clinical experience in the practice of marriage and family counseling, or a combination of 150 hours of approved supervision in the practice of psychotherapy that includes at least 50 hours of approved individual supervision in the practice of marriage and family counseling and 750 hours of supervised clinical experience in the practice of psychotherapy that includes at least 250 hours of clinical practice in marriage and family counseling. A person must pass a state licensing examination or the national examination for marriage and family therapists administered by the American Association of Marriage and Family Therapy Regulatory Boards, which is used as a licensure requirement in most states. Authorization under TRICARE requires licensing or certification in the state in which the provider practices.

TRICARE policy allows certified marriage and family therapists to provide covered services within their scope of licensure if they enter into a participation agreement (PA) to practice independently. A PA requires a provider to agree that a patient's physical health problems must receive appropriate concurrent management by a physician. If a PA is not signed, supervision and referral by a physician are required (*TRICARE Policy Manual* 6010.54-M, Chapter 11, Section 3.8, 2002).

## Pastoral Counselors

Pastoral counselors are trained in psychology and theology and provide counseling, as well as spiritual guidance, to patients. Certification by the American Association of Pastoral Counselors requires that people obtain a 3-year professional degree from a seminary and a specialized master's or doctoral degree in a mental health or behavioral health discipline. Postgraduate training includes at least 1,375 hours of supervised clinical experience and 250 hours of direct approved supervision (American Association of Pastoral Counselors, 2009).

Authorization under TRICARE requires licensure or certification by the state in which the counselor practices and a combination of 200 hours of approved supervision and 1,000 hours of supervised clinical experience in the practice of pastoral counseling or a combination of 150 hours of approved supervision in the practice of psychotherapy, including at least 50 hours of approved individual supervision in the practice of pastoral counseling, and 750 hours of supervised clinical experience in the practice of psychotherapy, with at least 250 hours of supervised clinical practice in pastoral counseling. As of 2009, six states licensed pastoral counselors: Arkansas, Kentucky, Maine, New Hampshire, North Carolina, and Tennessee. In states that do not offer licensure or certification, a pastoral counselor must be, or must meet all the requirements to become, a fellow or diplomate member in the American Association of Pastoral Counselors.

Pastoral counselors practicing under TRICARE must have a written referral and continuing supervision by a physician for their services to be reimbursable. However, because of the similarities among the requirements for licensure, certification, experience, and education, pastoral counselors may elect to be authorized as certified marriage and family therapists in many states and under TRICARE. That gives those providers the option of entering into a PA to practice independently under TRICARE. Without authorization as a marriage and family therapist and signing of a PA, services are covered only when a physician refers a beneficiary for therapy and continuing supervision by and communication with that physician is maintained throughout the course of treatment. Pastoral counselors cannot provide services under both provider categories (*TRICARE Policy Manual* 6010.54-M, Chapter 11, Section 3.9, 2002).

### Mental Health Counselors

Licensed mental health counselors (LMHCs) provide assessment and diagnosis of and treatment for mental illnesses, emotional problems, and substance-use issues to individuals and groups through psychotherapy, behavior modification, and counseling (AMHCA, 2009). Throughout the United States, several titles are used to identify people who practice in this discipline, including licensed professional counselor (LPC), licensed professional mental health counselor, licensed clinical professional counselor, licensed professional counselor of mental health, licensed clinical mental health counselor, and licensed mental health practitioner. *In this report, the term* counselor *is used generically to refer to these professionals; specific titles are used in the text when needed to conform to the terminology in specific publications that are being discussed.*

Educational requirements include a master's degree in mental health counseling or an allied mental health discipline from a graduate program in counseling and 2 years of post–master's degree clinical experience under the supervision of a licensed or certified mental health professional. Most states also require a minimum of 60 hours of graduate study and 3,000 hours of supervised experience to apply for licensure, but these criteria vary by state.

Under TRICARE policies, educational experience must include 3,000 hours of clinical work and 100 hours of face-to-face supervision. All counselors must pass a state or national licensure or certification examination to be considered authorized providers. If their state does not offer licensure to mental health counselors, they must be eligible for full clinical membership in the American Mental Health Counselors Association (AMHCA) or be certified as clinical mental health counselors by the Clinical Academy of the National Board of Certified Counselors (*TRICARE Policy Manual* 6010.54-M, Chapter 11, Section 3.10, 2002). Clinical membership in the AMHCA requires at least a master's degree in counseling from an accredited institution and a state license/certification or certification as a clinical mental health counselor (AMHCA, 2009). Counselors are not authorized to prescribe medication, and services rendered by them require referral and supervision by a physician to be reimbursed under TRICARE.

Referral and supervision requirements for mental health counselors[6] are delineated in 32 CFR § 199.6(c)(3)(iii)(K) and *TRICARE Policy Manual* 6010.54-M, Chapter 11, Section 3.1. They state that the services of these providers "may be provided only if the beneficiary is referred by a physician for the treatment of a medically diagnosed condition and a physician must also provide continuing and ongoing oversight and supervision of the program or episode of treatment" if they are to be considered for benefits on a fee-for-service basis. The terms of referral and supervision mandate that

- "Physicians must actually see the patient to evaluate and diagnose the condition to be treated prior to referring the beneficiary."
- "The referring physician [must provide] ongoing oversight of the course of referral related treatment throughout the period during which the beneficiary is being treated."
- "Written contemporaneous documentation of the referring physician's basis for referral and ongoing communication between the referring and treating provider regarding the oversight of the treatment rendered as a result of the referral must meet all requirements for medical records established by [the regulation]."

They also indicate that the "referring physician supervision does not require physical location on the premises of the treating provider or at the site of treatment."

Chapter 3 provides more detail on counselor's education, clinical training, and licensure and on the accreditation of institutions that grant their degrees.

## Mental Health Care by Primary-Care and Other Providers (Physicians, Advanced Practice Nurses, and Physician Assistants)

PCPs are physicians—typically general practitioners or family practitioners, internists, and pediatricians for younger patients—or physician assistants, nurse practitioners, or sometimes other health-care providers who are often patients' first point of contact with the health-

---

[6]These requirement also apply to persons practicing as pastoral counselors under TRICARE.

care system. Although they are not mental health specialists, they have a major role in differential diagnosis of and treatment for mental disorders, especially depression and anxiety. PCPs also typically play a part in managing patients' psychiatric symptoms in collaboration with mental health professionals (Kushner et al., 2001). Despite documented deficiencies in the quality of mental health care provided by PCPs, patients may prefer to see them or have few alternatives (Geller, 1999). Eaton and colleagues (2008) reported that military spouses most often received their mental health care from PCPs rather than from specialty mental health professionals.

PCPs may refer patients to counselors for treatment and supervise their work under the current TRICARE system.

## Other Specialists Not Recognized as Authorized Mental Health Providers

Substance-use counselors are not recognized in TRICARE as authorized mental health providers. Information on them is provided here because the committee's statement of task listed substance-use disorders among the health conditions of interest.

Substance-use counselors help people who have drug, alcohol, gambling, and food addictions to identify behaviors and problems related to their addictions. Most often, that counseling is done in a group setting, but it can also be done on an individual basis. The counselors also work with family members of people who have addictions and conduct programs aimed at preventing addiction (BLS, 2008-09c). The minimal educational requirements to qualify as a substance-use counselor are less rigorous than those for a mental health counselor. About half the states require a credential to practice, and more than half of these do not require a college degree. However, substance-use counselors are generally required to have about 1,000 hours more of supervised work experience than are mental health counselors. That is due in part to an apprentice training model adopted by the profession in which most of the knowledge, skills, and training is acquired through supervised experience on the job (Kerwin et al., 2006).

## ORIGIN OF THE STUDY

The issue of the independent practice of counselors has been discussed in Congress for several years. Various versions of several pieces of legislation—including the TRICARE Enhancement Act of 2000 (HR 4418, 106th Congress), the TRICARE Mental Health Services Enhancement Act (HR 2739, 107th Congress), the National Defense Authorization Act (NDAA) of Fiscal Year 2006 (HR 1815, 109th Congress), the NDAA for Fiscal Year 2007 (HR 5122, 109th Congress), and the NDAA for Fiscal Year 2008 (HR 1585, 110th Congress)—have proposed the expansion of counselors' responsibilities under TRICARE, including practice independent of physician referral and supervision. None of these proposals has been adopted into law.

### Summary and Review of *Expanding Access to Mental Health Counselors—Evaluation of the TRICARE Demonstration*

The 2001 NDAA directed DOD to implement a 1-year demonstration project in which access to qualified LMHCs was expanded by not requiring documentation of referral and supervision by a physician. The NDAA also required an evaluation of the demonstration's impact on service use, cost, and outcomes. As a result, TMA sponsored a study conducted by the Center for Military Health Policy Research (a joint venture of RAND Health and the RAND National Defense Institute) (Meredith et al., 2005). The demonstration project began on January 1, 2003. Mental health care utilization and outcomes were examined in the demonstration and comparison regions by analyzing data on claims before and after the demonstration and surveying beneficiaries after the demonstration. TMA chose two so-called catchment areas[7] in the TRICARE central region—Colorado Springs, Colorado, and Omaha, Nebraska—for the project "because their high volume of LMHCs would ensure ample providers for the demonstration" (Meredith et al., 2005, p. xiii).

---

[7]TRICARE defines a catchment area as follows: "the geographic area surrounding an MTF with inpatient capabilities. . . . Under TRICARE, a catchment area is also used as a planning tool to identify our eligible population, and define areas where our managed care support contractors must offer the TRICARE Prime benefit" (HA POLICY 97-038, March 5, 1997).

The RAND investigators hypothesized that the demonstration project might affect TRICARE beneficiaries and providers via

- Increased *access* to care delivered by mental health counselors resulting from fewer procedural barriers and less of a stigma from seeking counseling services, in contrast with no increased access to psychotropic medication care due to getting medicines solely from a doctor.
- Higher *utilization* of mental health services (especially counseling) as a function of direct access to LMHCs. There may be an increase in beneficiaries receiving both medication and counseling.
- Decreased total *cost* of care, again due to more use of mental health counselors (as a lower-cost alternative to other mental health specialists) and elimination of supervision costs.
- Increased or decreased *quality of care* among those seeing mental health counselors. Increased quality of care could be due to changes in professional roles, including greater autonomy and responsibility, earlier access to care, and earlier interventions. However, the demonstration could decrease quality of care through lower rates of collaboration with other professionals, especially for psychotropic medication treatment in collaboration with physicians, or through inappropriate visits, or based on some characteristics potentially associated with counselors (such as lower use of evidence-based therapy, lack of clinical skill to detect problems) (Meredith et al. 2005, pp. 9-10; emphasis in original).

The claims-data analyses found that in the overall beneficiary population, there was a small but statistically significant increase in the likelihood of being hospitalized for a psychiatric condition in the demonstration region. However, that the finding was not present in later analyses that controlled for characteristics of beneficiaries who were more likely to see LMHCs suggests that it was unrelated to LMHC care. In the overall beneficiary population, there was a decrease in the likelihood of seeing another mental health provider or non–mental health physician provider. In analyses that controlled for characteristics contributing to the likelihood of seeking services from an LMHC, beneficiaries who saw LMHCs were less likely to see psychiatrists and to receive psychotropic medication.[8] However, it is unknown whether those use changes were associated with differences in outcomes.

The survey data revealed that enrollees in the demonstration and comparison regions described no difference in access to mental health services, adherence to treatment, or mental health status. Enrollees in the demonstration region were more likely to report favorable ratings of counseling and treatment and of getting care when needed, although the cross-sectional nature of the survey design precludes determining whether this was a consequence of LMHC independent practice. Because the survey data were collected only after LMHC independent practice was implemented, it is possible that the results are due to regional differences and unrelated to the demonstration.

It is important to note that limitations in the data and study design preclude determining whether the LMHC independent practice resulted in different patient or beneficiary access to care or different outcomes. The demonstration project was conducted at roughly the same time as the initiation of major combat operations in Operation Iraqi Freedom. This mission has resulted in an increase in the demand for mental health care services in the active-duty military and their families, and the conclusions drawn regarding access may therefore not reflect current circumstances. Furthermore, even though the study found no evidence of changes in access to treatment as a result of the demonstration, the results might not be generalizable to regions where mental health providers are scarcer.

[8]Of note, unadjusted analyses indicated that a higher percentage of patients seen by LMHCs received psychotropic medication, compared to patients seeing other mental health counselors. However, that difference was observed in both the demonstration and the comparison regions (particularly before the demonstration, when all LMHCs were required to have supervision and referral by a physician). The difference probably reflects preceding referral or supervision requirements rather than being evidence of prescribing patterns of LMHCs versus other mental health providers if supervision or referral requirements were similar. Furthermore, the observation that, in unadjusted analyses, psychotropic-medication use among patients seeing LMHCs declined by nearly 11% in the demonstration area and 3% in the comparison area suggests that the unadjusted results are consistent with the adjusted (i.e., patients seeing LMHCs have a lower likelihood of receiving psychotropic medication than those seeing other mental health providers).

## Department of Defense Response to Congressional Inquiries Regarding the Use of Counselors in the Military Health System

DOD submitted the RAND study to Congress on May 10, 2005. About 6 months later, a House conference report that accompanied the FY 2006 National Defense Authorization Act (US Congress, House of Representatives, 2005) directed DOD to produce a report that included a review of the quality of care provided by LMHCs in the Military Health System (MHS) (DOD, 2006).

The resulting report—*Aspects of the Use of Licensed Professional Counselors in the Military Health System. Report to Congress* (DOD, 2006)—was delivered in June 2006. It offers insights into DOD's concerns regarding the independent practice of counselors (referred to as LPCs in the text), which were summarized in the text (pp. 9-10) as follows:

> There remains significant variability among the states in training programs and requirements for licensure as a mental health counselor. . . . Some counselors attend training programs accredited by the CACREP,[9] a nationally recognized accrediting agency, while many do not. In most states a qualifying education requires only minimal coursework in diagnosis and treatment of mental disorders and no specific clinical experience with individuals with mental disorders. In some states licensure as a professional counselor can be obtained with a Masters-level postgraduate degree in fields only "related" to counseling. While there is evidence that the extent of training variability has decreased over time, it remains a reality that professional counselors licensed to practice have an unevenness of exposure to classroom education and supervised clinical experiences in the assessment and treatment of persons with mental disorders.

The report states (p. 10) that the purpose of the current policy of supervision of counselors is to "ensure that the quality of care provided to our beneficiaries is not compromised by differences in scope of training and experience from other currently authorized groups of providers." However, it stipulates that physician oversight of counselors' clinical

[9]The Council on Accreditation of Counseling and Related Educational Programs (CACREP) accredits graduate-level counselor-education programs. CACREP's function and requirements are addressed extensively in Chapter 4.

work "occurs predominantly on paper" and is "difficult to ensure to any great degree" (p. 9).

The report notes that "quality of care for mental health . . . in the MHS is determined largely by the credentialing process and application for TRICARE provider status." It gives as an example the Navy's use of counselors in its Fleet and Family Support Programs (FFSPs)[10] in states in which counselors are authorized to practice independently. In these circumstances, providers are granted practice privileges on a case-by-case basis , using a standard that specifies education, training, and experience requirements (SECNAVINST 1754.7A; the standard is discussed in greater detail in Chapter 3). The report indicates (p. 8) that

> when using the strict criteria . . . to privilege LPC providers, Navy FFSPs have not noted any consistent differences in the quality of care provided by LPCs when compared to other Master's-level practitioners. Similarly, no qualitative differences in care are noted by health care administrators operating in the TRICARE managed care system.

It concludes that "referral to LPCs has been strengthened through the use of primary care physicians as the referral source" but that

> given the practical obstacles to physician supervision of LPCs and the perceived impediment to accessing services caused by the physician referral requirement, it would be prudent to explore issues of supervision, referral, provider credentialing, and scope of practice to develop options that would preserve quality of care, safeguard the health and well-being of Service members and maximize access to mental health care for all beneficiaries.

## The National Defense Authorization Act for Fiscal Year 2008 Directive

The NDAA for Fiscal Year 2008 (Public Law 110-181) directed DOD to enter into a contract with IOM "for the purpose of (1) conducting an independent study of the credentials, preparation, and training of individuals practicing as licensed mental health counselors;

---

[10]FFSPs provide a variety of support services to Navy personnel and their families, including employment, financial, relocation, transition, and counseling assistance; they are not medical-care facilities.

and (2) making recommendations for permitting licensed mental health counselors to practice independently under the TRICARE program." In response to that mandate and to fulfill the resulting contract, IOM formed the Committee on the Qualifications of Professionals Providing Mental Health Counseling Services Under TRICARE in early 2009.

## COMMITTEE STATEMENT OF TASK

DOD specified several elements for the committee to address:

- **Educational requirements**—The report shall provide for an assessment of the educational requirements and curricula relevant to mental health practice for licensed mental health counselors, including types of degrees recognized, certification standards for graduate programs for such profession, and recognition of undergraduate coursework for completion of graduate degree requirements and the extent to which such educational requirements prepare licensed mental health counselors to diagnose and treat such illness such as major depressive disorder, schizophrenia, post-traumatic stress disorder, bipolar disorder, mental disorders due to a general medical condition, somatoform disorders and delirium, dementia, amnestic, substance use and other disorders regularly associated with head trauma.
- **Licensing requirements**—The report shall provide for an assessment of State licensing requirements for licensed mental health counselors, including for each level of licensure if a State issues more than one type of license for the profession. The assessment shall examine requirements in the areas of education, training, examination, continuing education, and ethical standards, and shall include an evaluation of the extent to which States authorize members of the licensed mental health counselor profession to diagnose and treat mental illnesses, including illness such as major depressive disorder, schizophrenia, post-traumatic stress disorder, bipolar disorder, mental disorders due to a general medical condition, somatoform disorders and delirium, dementia, amnestic, substance use and other disorders regularly associated with head trauma.
- **Clinical experience requirements**—The report shall provide for an analysis of the requirements for clinical experience for a licensed mental health counselor to be recognized under regulations for the TRICARE program, and the extent to which such

clinical experience requirements prepare licensed mental health counselors to diagnose and treat such illness such [sic] as major depressive disorder, schizophrenia, post-traumatic stress disorder, bipolar disorder, mental disorders due to a general medical condition, somatoform disorders and delirium, dementia, amnestic, substance use and other disorders regularly associated with head trauma, and recommendations, if any, for standardization or adjustment of such requirements.

- **Independent practice under other federal programs**—The report shall provide for an assessment of the extent to which licensed mental health counselors are authorized to practice independently under other Federal programs (such as the Medicare program, the Department of Veterans Affairs, the Indian Health Service, and Head Start), and a review of the relationship, if any, between recognition of mental health professions under the Medicare program and independent practice authority for such profession under the TRICARE program.
- **Independent practice under FEHBP**—The report shall provide for an assessment of the extent to which licensed mental health counselors are authorized to practice independently under the Federal Employee Health Benefits Program and private insurance plans. The assessment shall identify the States having laws requiring private insurers to cover, or offer coverage of, the services of members of licensed mental health counselors and shall identify the conditions, if any, that are placed on coverage of practitioners under the profession by insurance plans and how frequently these types of conditions are used by insurers.
- **Historical review of regulations**—The report shall provide for a review of the history of regulations prescribed by the Department of Defense regarding which members of the mental health profession are recognized as providers under the TRICARE program as independent practitioners, whether such regulations and/or other applicable policies were at the direction of Congress, and an examination of the recognition by the Department of third-party certification for members of such profession.
- **Clinical exposure and capabilities studies**—The report shall include a review and synthesis of available data describing the proportion of all patients under the care of licensed mental health counselors with major depressive disorder, schizophrenia, post-traumatic stress disorder, bipolar disorder, mental disorders due to a general medical condition, somatoform disorders and delirium, dementia, amnestic, substance use and other disorders

regularly associated with head trauma. Additionally, the report shall include a review of outcome studies and of the literature regarding the comparative quality and effectiveness of care provided by licensed mental health counselors, particularly with respect to effectiveness of care for persons with major depressive disorder, schizophrenia, post-traumatic stress disorder, bipolar disorder, mental disorders due to a general medical condition, somatoform disorders and delirium, dementia, amnestic, substance use and other disorders regularly associated with head trauma and provide an independent review of the findings.

- **Conclusions and recommendations**—The report shall include conclusions and recommendations for permitting licensed mental health counselors to practice independently under the TRICARE program including recommendation regarding modifications of current policy for the TRICARE program with respect to allowing licensed mental health counselors to practice independently in the TRICARE program, paying particular attention to the preparedness of licensed mental health counselors to diagnose, treat and appropriately refer persons with disorders of particular importance to TRICARE beneficiaries including major depressive disorder, post-traumatic stress disorder, mental disorders due to a general medical condition, somatoform disorders and delirium, dementia, amnestic, substance use and other disorders regularly associated with head trauma.
- **Limitations to practice**—The report shall include any recommendations [regarding] limitations to practice independently with respect to DOD beneficiaries.

DOD did not ask for an analysis of issues surrounding access to mental health care. As already noted, that was the central topic of the 2005 RAND monograph *Expanding Access to Mental Health Counselors—Evaluation of the TRICARE Demonstration* (Meredith et al., 2005). Access to care was also discussed in a 2007 report by the DOD Task Force on Mental Health. That report found that "mental health professionals are not sufficiently accessible to service members" and that children of service members and members of the National Guard and Reserve experience particularly constrained access. The task force recommended that DOD "ensure a full continuum of care to support psychological health is available and accessible to all service members and their eligible family members, regardless of location" and recommended changes to TRICARE's resources, staffing, number of providers, and care obligations to accomplish it.

## COMMITTEE APPROACH TO TASK

To answer the questions posed by the sponsor, the committee undertook a wide-ranging evaluation of the scientific literature, relevant laws and regulations, and publications produced by mental health professionals and educational and other organizations affiliated with them.

Data sources and keyword searches were selected according to their overall relevance to the topic of interest. Because of the interdisciplinary nature of the topic, a wide array of electronic databases were queried, including PsycINFO and PsycARTICLES. To supplement the computerized searches, the reference sections of related and relevant publications were searched manually. General and specialized Internet search engines were used to find references in fields not covered by scholarly databases.

The committee also benefited from presentations by the sponsor, professional organizations, managed-care providers, and experts in various relevant issues during two workshops. Appendix A lists the participants and their topics. Many of the organizations and individuals provided additional information for the committee's consideration and responded to questions and requests for data. Their efforts greatly aided the committee's work.

## OVERVIEW OF RELATED INSTITUTE OF MEDICINE REPORTS

IOM has published several reports that address issues relevant to the present subject, in particular the delivery of mental health services to and mental health issues in military populations. They are summarized briefly below. Some reports are revisited in greater detail in the chapters that follow.

### IOM Studies Addressing the Delivery of Mental Health Services

The IOM committee responsible for *Managing Managed Care: Quality Improvement in Behavioral Health* (IOM, 1997) was charged with developing a framework for performance indicators, accreditation standards, and quality-improvement mechanisms that could be used for managed behavioral health care. The report concluded that multiple players—including local, state, and federal governments; accreditation, managed-care, purchaser, professional, and consumer organizations; and the mass media—are involved in quality assessment, but information for informed purchasing decisions is lacking. It recommended that quality of care be monitored with relevant performance measures, valid accreditation processes, evidence-based outcome measures, and clinical practice guidelines. It further recommended that quality be clearly addressed in contracts between purchasers and providers, and it suggested that federal and state governments encourage the development of report cards and include all stakeholders in developing, implementing, and using consumer-protection standards.

The goal of *Crossing the Quality Chasm: A New Health System for the 21st Century* (IOM, 2001) was to identify strategies to improve the quality of US health care substantially. The report concluded that all health-care organizations, professional groups, and purchasers should strive for health care that is safe, effective, patient-centered, timely, efficient, and equitable. A 21st-century health-care delivery system, it said, should have health-care processes that are based on continuous healing relationships, shared information between clinicians and patients, evidence-based decision making, and collaboration among clinicians and institutions. The report recommended restructuring clinical education and assessing provider credentialing to be consistent with those health-system principles. It also recommended applying work-design principles that are used in other industries, using information technology to support decision making, and realigning payment policies to improve quality of care.

A later report—*Improving the Quality of Health Care for Mental and Substance-Use Conditions: Quality Chasm Series* (IOM, 2006a)—examined whether the *Quality Chasm* approach was relevant to health care for mental and substance-use (M/SU) conditions. It concluded that the framework is applicable to behavioral health care and that improving US health care overall requires attending to M/SU health-care quality issues and delivering care with an understanding of mind–body interactions. The report recommended that M/SU clinicians and organizations use process and outcome measures to improve the quality of care. It also recommended the development of national standards for credentialing and licensure of M/SU providers that are based on specific clinical competencies.

## IOM Studies Addressing Mental Health Issues in Military Populations

As part of a larger research effort on veterans' health issues, IOM committees have been working on a series of reports on the effects of psychological stress on present and former members of the military. Among them is the 2006 report *Posttraumatic Stress Disorder: Diagnosis and Assessment* (IOM, 2006b), which provided responses to a series of questions posed by the Department of Veterans Affairs, the report's sponsor. They included, What constitutes optimal evaluation of a patient for PTSD? and What neuropsychological evaluation or other testing should be included in an optimal evaluation of a patient for PTSD? The report concluded that PTSD is a disorder that has robust core clinical features that are consistent among diverse populations. It strongly recommended that PTSD be diagnosed through a face-to-face clinical interview by a health professional trained in diagnosing psychiatric disorders. The report did not draw specific conclusions regarding the training of mental health professionals who perform the diagnosis and assessment.

A later report in the series—*Treatment of Posttraumatic Stress Disorder: An Assessment of the Evidence* (IOM, 2008b)—reviewed and assessed the evidence on the efficacy of pharmacological and psychological treatment for PTSD. It sought not to develop clinical practice recommendations but to reach evidence-based conclusions that would inform policy decisions. The committee responsible for the report concluded that the evidence existing when it completed its work was inadequate to determine the efficacy of any pharmacotherapy in the treatment of PTSD.[11] It found that the evidence was sufficient to conclude that exposure therapy, a form of cognitive-behavioral therapy, was effective in the treatment of PTSD. There was insufficient evidence to draw conclusions on other psychotherapy, including eye-movement desensitization and reprocessing therapy, cognitive restructuring, coping-skills training, and therapy delivered in group formats.

The 2008 report *Gulf War and Health, Volume 6: Physiologic, Psychologic, and Psychosocial Effects of Deployment-Related Stress* (IOM, 2008a) concluded that there is a consistent, positive association between deployment and specific health effects, such as psychiatric disorders (including

---

[11]The committee did *not* conclude that pharmacotherapy was ineffective but rather that the evidence base was insufficient.

PTSD, other anxiety disorders, and depressive disorders), alcohol abuse, accidental death or suicide in the early years after deployment, and marital and family conflict. It also concluded there is limited but suggestive evidence of an association between deployment and incarceration or drug abuse. Finally, it reported inadequate or insufficient evidence to determine whether there is a relationship between deployment and neurocognitive and neurobehavioral effects, sleep disorders or disturbance, homelessness, or adverse employment outcomes. The report recommended that DOD conduct predeployment and postdeployment screenings for medical conditions and psychosocial status to identify at-risk personnel, implement interventions, and measure long-term consequences of deployment.

### Other IOM Studies

In 2009, IOM released *Redesigning Continuing Education in the Health Professions*. This report concluded that there are major flaws in the way continuing education (CE) for medical professionals in the United States is conducted, financed, regulated, and evaluated. It found that CE differs widely among and within health professions in terms of content and delivery or learning methods and that it is largely driven by state requirements and regulatory bodies that often focus on the number of hours spent in CE courses. It concluded that requirements that are based on credit hours rather than outcomes—and that vary by state and profession—are not conducive to teaching and maintaining core competencies aimed at providing quality care. The report suggests a new vision for CE based on an approach called "continuing professional development," in which learning takes place over a lifetime and stretches beyond the classroom to the point of care. It also recommends that consideration be given to creating a national independent institute that would focus on improving CE regulation, including accreditation, certification, credentialing, and licensure.

## ORGANIZATION OF THIS REPORT

The remainder of this report is organized into five chapters and supporting appendixes. Chapter 2 provides background information on the characteristics of the TRICARE beneficiary population and some of the mental health issues that they face. Chapter 3 describes how counselors are trained and practice and contrasts this with training and practice of other mental health professionals; the chapter also delineates educational, licensing, and clinical experience requirements for counselors and examines the accreditation of the educational institutions that train them and the examinations that they must pass to enter professional practice. Chapter 4 addresses how counselors practice in other programs that are under the aegis of the federal government. Research regarding the delivery of high-quality mental health care is reviewed in Chapter 5 with a focus on psychosocial services relevant to conditions found in the TRICARE enrollee population. Chapter 6 compiles the report's findings and offers overall conclusions and recommendations.

Agendas from the public meetings held by the committee are provided in Appendix A. Appendix B provides excerpts from the section of the CFR that delineates the rules governing the practice of authorized mental health providers under TRICARE. Working definitions of some key terms used in the report are presented in Appendix C. Appendix D presents excerpts of salient sections of the *United States Code* that describe the scope of practice and the training, experience, and licensing requirements imposed on mental health professionals who practice in the TRICARE system. Excerpts of the regulation that defines the scope of practice and supervision requirements for licensed counselors in the US Army are presented in Appendix E. Appendix F presents a clinical vignette that is intended to provide insight into the complexities of cases that a TRICARE mental health practitioner may face. A comprehensive list of licensing requirements for counselors in the United States is contained in Appendix G. Appendix H provides biographic information on the committee members, consultants, and staff responsible for this study.

## REFERENCES

AADPRT (American Association of Directors of Psychiatric Residency Training). 2009. *What is psychiatry training?* http://www.aadprt.org/training/default.aspx. (Accessed November 5, 2009).

American Association for Marriage and Family Therapy. 2009. *FAQ's on MFT's.* http://www.aamft.org/faqs/index_nm.asp. (Accessed November 5, 2009).

American Association of Pastoral Counselors. 2009. *About pastoral counseling.* http://www.aapc.org/content/about-pastoral-counseling. (Accessed November 5, 2009).

American Nurses Credentialing Center. 2009. *Clinical nurse specialist in adult psychiatric & mental health certification eligibility criteria.* http://www.nursecredentialing.org/Eligibility/AdultPsychMentalHealthCNSEligibility.aspx. (Accessed November 5, 2009).

AMHCA (American Mental Health Counselors Association). 2009. *American Mental Health Counselors Association.* http://www.amhca.org/. (Accessed November 5, 2009).

APA (American Psychological Association). 2009. *About clinical psychology.* http://www.apa.org/divisions/div12/aboutcp.html. (Accessed November 5, 2009).

BLS (Bureau of Labor Statistics). 2008-09a. Psychologists. In *Occupational outlook handbook,* 2008-09 ed. http://www.bls.gov/oco/ocos056.htm. (Accessed November 5, 2009).

BLS. 2008-09b. Social workers. In *Occupational outlook handbook,* 2008-09 ed. http://www.bls.gov/oco/ocos060.htm. (Accessed November 5, 2009).

BLS. 2008-09c. Counselors. In *Occupational outlook handbook,* 2008-09 ed. http://www.bls.gov/oco/ocos067.htm. (Accessed November 5, 2009).

DOD (Department of Defense). 2006. *Aspects of the use of licensed professional counselors in the Military Health System. Report to Congress.* Transmittal letter, August 28. http://www.tricare.mil/planning/congress/downloads/2006/new/Licensed-Mental.pdf. (Accessed October 20, 2009).

DOD. 2007. *An achievable vision: Report of the Department of Defense Task Force on Mental Health.* Falls Church, VA: Defense Health Board. www.health.mil/dhb/mhtf/MHTF-Report-Final.pdf. (Accessed October 27, 2009).

DOD. 2009. Who we are & our history. In *TRICARE fundamentals course,* Section 14, Participant guide. http://www.tricare.mil/tricareu/docs/200906/14_Who_We_Are_June_09.doc. (Accessed September 18, 2009).

Eaton KM, Hoge CW, Messer SC, Whitt AA, Cabrera OA, McGurk D, Cox A, Castro CA. 2008. Prevalence of mental health problems, treatment need, and barriers to care among primary care-seeking spouses of military service members involved in Iraq and Afghanistan deployments. *Military Medicine* 173(11):1051-1056.

Geller JM. 1999. Rural primary care providers' perceptions of their roles in the provision of mental health services: Voices from the plains. *Journal of Rural Health* 15(3):326-334.

HHS (Department of Health and Human Services). 2009. *Guidelines for mental health HPSA designation.* Health Resources and Services Administration. http://bhpr.hrsa.gov/shortage/hpsaguidement.htm. (Accessed November 13, 2009).

IOM (Institute of Medicine). 1997. *Managing managed care: Quality improvement in behavioral health.* Washington DC: National Academy Press.

IOM. 2001. *Crossing the quality chasm: A new health system for the 21st century.* Washington, DC: National Academy Press.

IOM. 2006a. *Improving the quality of health care for mental and substance-use conditions: Quality chasm series.* Washington, DC: The National Academies Press.

IOM. 2006b. *Posttraumatic stress disorder: Diagnosis and assessment.* Washington, DC: The National Academies Press.

IOM. 2008a. *Gulf War and health, Volume 6: Physiologic, psychologic, and psychosocial effects of deployment-related stress.* Washington, DC: The National Academies Press.

IOM. 2008b. *Treatment of posttraumatic stress disorder: An assessment of the evidence.* Washington, DC: The National Academies Press.

IOM. 2009. *Redesigning continuing education in the health professions.* Washington, DC: The National Academies Press.

Kerwin ME, Walker-Smith K, Kirby KC. 2006. Comparative analysis of state requirements for the training of substance abuse and mental health counselors. *Journal of Substance Abuse Treatment* 30(3):173-181.

Kushner K, Diamond R, Beasley JW, Mundt M, Plane MB, Robbins K. 2001. Primary care physicians' experience with mental health consultation. *Psychiatric Services* 52(6):838-840.

Meredith LS, Tanielian T, Greenberg MD, Suarez A, Eiseman E. 2005. *Expanding access to mental health counselors: Evaluation of the TRICARE demonstration.* Santa Monica, CA: RAND Corporation.

NQMC (National Quality Measures Clearinghouse). 2005. *Guidance on TRICARE standards/regulations: Qualified mental health professionals scope of practice & supervision.* Agency for Healthcare Research and Quality, U.S. Department of Health and Human Services. http://www.maximus.com/nqmc/downloads/Qualified_Mental_Health_Professional.doc. (Accessed October 25, 2009).

OPM (U.S. Office of Personnel Management). 2009. Creditable service for leave accrual. In *The guide to processing personnel actions.* http://www.opm.gov/Feddata/gppa/Gppa06.pdf. (Accessed October 29, 2009).

Ralph JA, Sammons MT. 2006. Future directions in miltary psychology. In *Military psychology: Clinical and operational applications,* edited by Kennedy CH and Zillmer EA. New York: Guilford. Pp. 371-386.

*Stars and Stripes.* 2009. Six million beneficiaries to get new TRICARE contractors. Pacific edition, July 18. http://www.stripes.com/article.asp?section=140&article=63754. (Accessed October 10, 2009).

TRICARE Policy Manual 6010.54-M, Chapter 11, Addendum A(2)(B). 2002. *Participation agreement for partial hospitalization program services.* http://www.tricare.mil/tp02/C11ADA.PDF. (Accessed November 13, 2009).

TRICARE Policy Manual 6010.54-M, Chapter 11, Section 3.5. 2002. *Certified clinical social worker.* http://www.tricare.mil/TP02/C11S3_5.PDF. (Accessed November 13, 2009).

TRICARE Policy Manual 6010.54-M, Chapter 11, Section 3.6. 2002. *Certified psychiatric nurse specialist.* http://www.tricare.mil/TP02/C11S3_6.PDF. (Accessed November 13, 2009).

TRICARE Policy Manual 6010.54-M, Chapter 11, Section 3.7. 2002. *Clinical psychologist.* http://www.tricare.mil/TP02/C11S3_7.PDF. (Accessed November 13, 2009).

TRICARE Policy Manual 6010.54-M, Chapter 11, Section 3.8. 2002. *Certified marriage and family therapist.* http://www.tricare.mil/TP02/C11S3_8.PDF. (Accessed November 13, 2009).

TRICARE Policy Manual 6010.54-M, Chapter 11, Section 3.9. 2002. *Pastoral counselor.* http://www.tricare.mil/TP02/C11S3_9.PDF. (Accessed November 13, 2009).

TRICARE Policy Manual 6010.54-M, Chapter 11, Section 3.10. 2002. *Mental health counselor.* http://www.tricare.mil/TP02/C11S3_10.PDF. (Accessed November 13, 2009).

TRICARE. 2009a. *TRICARE Behavioral health care services.* Brochure, July. http://www.tricare.mil/mybenefit/Download/Forms/BHC_Flyer_09_L.pdf. (Accessed October 10, 2009).

TRICARE. 2009b. *TRICARE beneficiary handbook*. http://www.tricare.mil/tricaresmartfiles/Prod_125/BW_HB_LO_RES.pdf. (Accessed October 10, 2009). Note that several versions of this handbook are extant, addressing different regions and specific programs. An online version of this information is also available: http://www.tricare.mil/mybenefit/.

US Congress, House of Representatives. 2005. *Report 109-360. National Defense Authorization Act for Fiscal Year 2006. Conference report to accompany H.R. 1815. 109th Congress, 1st Session,* December 18. http://frwebgate.access.gpo.gov/cgi-bin/getdoc.cgi?dbname=109_cong_reports&docid=f:hr360.109.pdf. (Accessed October 5, 2009).

# 2

# TRICARE Beneficiaries and Mental Health Issues in Military Families

This chapter addresses the characteristics of the TRICARE beneficiary population and the mental health issues that they face. It begins with a brief summary of the demographics of the population and a discussion of their special exposures, risk factors, and protective factors. Information on mental health disorders follows, focusing on the conditions identified in the committee's statement of task and on psychosocial issues for US military families. The chapter concludes with a presentation of data on patients under the care of counselors.

The intent of the chapter is to provide background information on patients that might be seen by mental health professionals who deliver diagnostic and treatment services to TRICARE beneficiaries.

## DEMOGRAPHICS OF THE TRICARE POPULATION

TRICARE submits yearly reports of its operations to Congress that include details on the demographics of its beneficiary population. That information is summarized below.

In 2008, TRICARE served a population of 9.4 million beneficiaries (TRICARE, 2009). The 8.8 million who reside or are stationed in the United States are divided into three regions—North, South, and West—that provide care to roughly equal proportions of that population (HealthNet Federal Services, 2009; Humana Military Healthcare

Services, 2009; TriWest, 2009). The remaining beneficiaries—about 0.6 million—are covered in overseas regions.

Only about 20% of beneficiaries are active-duty members of the armed forces or activated members of the National Guard or Reserves; 26% are family members (including children) of active-duty or activated personnel, and 54% are retirees and their families (TRICARE, 2009). Almost half the beneficiaries are female (48.5%). Figure 2.1 shows the beneficiary population's age diversity.

Appendix B contains additional demographic and socioeconomic information about the general military population (including families) and the Operation Iraqi Freedom (OIF) and Operation Enduring Freedom (OEF) warfighters. The data there are intended to provide more background on the similarities and differences between the TRICARE population and other managed–health-care populations.

## SPECIAL EXPOSURES AND RISK FACTORS IN THE TRICARE POPULATION

Military life presents a number of exposures and risk factors that may influence the likelihood of experiencing a mental health problem. Different factors affect different segments of the beneficiary population. They are discussed below to highlight some of the issues that must be considered in evaluating the readiness of practitioners to provide diagnoses to and treat the population.

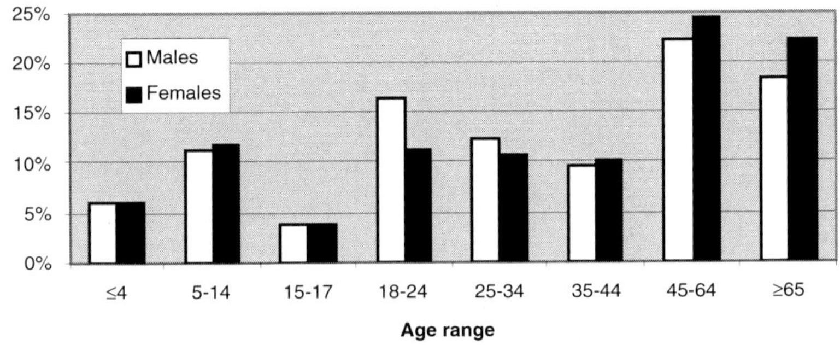


**FIGURE 2.1** Age distribution of the TRICARE beneficiary population.
NOTE: Percentages shown are percentages for each sex, not the whole beneficiary population.
SOURCE: TRICARE (2009).

## Combat Exposure and Traumatic Stressors

Combat exposure is one of the greatest stressors that a person can experience. In theater, combat veterans report frequent encounters with roadside improvised explosive devices (IEDs), suicide bombers, snipers, and an omnipresent insurgence characterized by an inability to differentiate combatants from noncombatants. Patrol operations may entail attacking, being attacked, killing, and witnessing mutilations and other carnage. OIF and OEF troops report distress over ethical violations to be a central problem (MHAT, 2006). Although most soldiers and marines reported receiving adequate battlefield-ethics training, over one-fourth reported encountering situations in which they did not know how to respond (MHAT, 2006). Feelings of helplessness and guilt may fuel the experience of emotional turmoil and depression. Multiple deployments, longer deployments, and the constancy of a 24/7 threatening living environment characterize tours of duty. A state of anxiety interferes with sleep (a major protective factor in survival) and erodes resilience.

A sample of service members who had been deployed to OIF or OEF reported exposure to a wide array of traumatic events; 50% noted that they had a friend who was killed or seriously wounded, and 45% saw people who were dead or seriously wounded (Tanielian and Jaycox, 2008). In a study conducted by Hoge et al. (2004), 2,586 Army and 815 Marine Corps combat infantry troops were interviewed and completed postdeployment surveys. During their tours of duty in Iraq, 92% were attacked or ambushed; 95% received small arms fire; 94% saw dead bodies or human remains; 89% received artillery, rocket, or mortar fire; 86% knew someone who was killed or seriously injured; and 56% reported being responsible for the death of an enemy combatant.

Research indicates that TRICARE may experience a relatively high volume of OIF and OEF veterans seeking treatment for posttraumatic stress disorder (PTSD) in the coming years. A team of researchers with the San Francisco Department of Veterans Affairs (VA) Medical Center discovered a time lag in reporting of mental health problems among OIF and OEF veterans—up to 2 years postservice (Seal et al., 2009). The data point to a need for providers, not only in the VA system but in TRICARE, to be prepared for waves of OIF and OEF veterans and their family members seeking mental health and psychosocial services. Research findings generated by Charles Hoge and his team at the Walter Reed Army Medical Center Research Center suggest that spouses manifest rates of mental health problems similar to those in soldiers; TRICARE probably also needs to be prepared to respond to mental health issues presented by family members (Eaton et al., 2008).

Active-duty servicewomen face some unique experiences during their deployments. They participate in a wide array of duties and have experienced comparable exposure to combat (IOM, 2008). Female service members face issues related specifically to physical violence, sexual harassment, and assault. Over the last 2 decades, there has been increasing attention to violence and sexist harassment against female service members. The emphasis on strong masculine traits, the war culture, the devaluing of feminine traits, and sexual slurs increase the risk of victimization of women (Donohoe, 2005). In a convenience sample of 270 female veterans, 33% reported experiencing a sexual assault during their service in the military (Surís et al., 2004). Women who reported rape or dual victimization (both rape and other forms of violence) were more likely also to report chronic health problems, prescription drug use for emotional problems, failure to complete college, and annual income less than $25,000. Women who reported dual traumas also reported the most severe impairment (Sadler et al., 2000). In a more recent study conducted by Street et al. (2008), the coinvestigators discovered a high prevalence of sexual harassment and assault and rates higher among female service members. Such victimization was associated with not only more immediate physical and mental health effects but long-term health-care needs. Higher rates of PTSD in women are statistically associated with increasing rates of military sexual assault. In a meta-analysis of 21 papers, Goldzweig et al. (2006) reported rates of sexual harassment of 55–99% and rates of sexual assault of 4.2–7.3% in active-duty women compared with 11–48% in female veterans. The noteworthy disparity in reported rates can be partially explained by victimized active-duty soldiers' fear of retaliation, especially if the offenders were superior officers or if allegations had been countered with censure.

## Issues for Military Families and Retirees

Demographic data compiled by the Department of Defense (DOD, 2007a) show that 57.7% of active-duty service members have family responsibilities; that is, they have spouses, one or more children, or other dependents. The demographic profile of Reserve and National Guard families is similar.

As in society at large, the health of a military family is influenced by the health of the service member, and the health and productivity of the service member are integrally related to and enhanced by the health and welfare of the family. Military occupation and duties involve a variety of stressors. They include a mobile lifestyle, isolation from the civilian community and extended family, adjustment to the rules and regulations of military life, and frequent family separations due to frequent deployments. In addition, stressors for female spouses are complicated by worries about jobs, child rearing, and household duties while male service members are deployed. Along similar lines, the male partner of a deployed female service member may encounter difficulties in adjusting to new roles in caretaking and management of the home. For single mothers, added stress is related to the enlisting of family members, friends, or hired child-care workers to provide care for their children during deployment. In general, if the nondeployed civilian partner of a service member finds military life stressful or unsatisfactory, the service member also becomes dissatisfied and more likely to leave the military (Eaton et al., 2008). Eaton and colleagues found, in their study of 940 spouses of service members deployed to Iraq or Afghanistan, that spouses reported types and magnitudes of mental health problems similar to those of the service members and that spouses were more likely to seek mental health services for those problems. Spouses did not seem to be as concerned about the stigma of mental health care as service members. Spouses most often sought and received care from their primary-care physicians; this may be related to the lack of mental health services for spouses on military installations. A DOD Task Force on Mental Health report indicated that mental health services for spouses are not adequately provided through the TRICARE insurance network (DOD, 2007b).

Much attention has been given to the needs of service members and spouses, but many military families are concerned about having adequate mental health resources for their children, especially school-age and adolescent youth. Parental concerns expressed, in addition to facilitating typical childhood development, include parenting skills to manage frequent deployments, reintegration and reentry programs when the service member returns to the family, addressing anxiety and fears experienced by children with regard to the deployed parent, managing multiple moves, and bereavement support (National Military Family Association, 2006).

Retirees make up a substantial portion of the TRICARE beneficiary population. Many of them are also veterans. Among the veterans seeking care, depression is one of the most common chronic conditions treated in VA Medical Centers (Cully et al., 2008). That may be the result of untreated mental health conditions incurred during military service or independent of military service. Retirees may be coping with the loss of a spouse or managing chronic or long-term illness other than mental health problems. Other studies have shown that veterans have higher rates of alcohol misuse, which is often associated with depression (IOM, 2008).

## Risk Factors

The greatest risk factors for mental health problems during deployment include higher intensity of exposure to combat stressors; greater length of deployment; female sex; lower socioeconomic status; lower rank; absence of peer, social, and family supports; and a history of childhood trauma[1] (IOM, 2008).

One major risk factor associated with the onset of PTSD is physical injury. In a study of returning OIF veterans conducted by Hoge et al. (2007), those who were physically injured had 3 times as great a risk of developing PTSD, regardless of the severity of the injury, as the non-injured. The incidence of PTSD increases significantly with the number of injuries suffered.

Rates of PTSD and major depression were highest among Army soldiers, Marines, and those who were no longer on active duty (people in the Reserves and those discharged or retired from the military). Women, Hispanics, and enlisted personnel were more likely to report symptoms of PTSD and major depression; the best predictor of these conditions was exposure to combat (Tanielian and Jaycox, 2008).

## Protective Factors

Many service members arrive home fortified by their resilience and reintegrate into their communities without adverse mental health effects. Pride and a sense of accomplishment often prevail. In consid-

---

[1]In contrast, however, Yehuda and colleagues report that managing the legacies of childhood traumatic events provides a combat soldier with a sense of protective mastery and efficacy (Yehuda et al., 2006).

ering resilience, it is important to recognize the important influences of protective factors that mediate the effects of adverse events. First, *constitutional hardiness* often refers to the "healthy-soldier effect" based on physical fitness and psychological readiness to assume an assertive, active, coping style. Second, during all phases of the deployment cycle, service members who have experienced the most comprehensive training, strong leadership, unit cohesion, and an esprit de corps are buffered against adverse health effects. In reservists and members of the National Guard, in particular, navigating assignments to a new unit and establishing new connections may undermine resilience. Third, a validating and supportive homecoming is also important. Research points to the centrality of family and social supports as major protective factors (Friedman, 2006). The social supports include loved ones; immediate-family and extended-family members; work colleagues; members of a church, mosque, or temple; support networks for military partners and families; and a wide array of health-care and mental health–care providers. Such positive social supports serve as vital buffers against the emergence of mental health problems.

## "Signature" Mental Health and Psychosocial Issues

Unlike Vietnam-era veterans, for whom PTSD was the prominent adverse mental health outcome, veterans of recent conflicts report high rates of various distinct yet interrelated syndromes, including PTSD, depression with suicidal ideation and behavior, substance misuse and abuse, and traumatic brain injury (TBI). Milliken and colleagues (2009) found that when service members who had returned from Iraq were rescreened about 6 months after an initial assessment, they reported more adverse mental health concerns and were referred for care at significantly higher rates; this suggests that some problems take time to manifest after deployment.

A 2008 Institute of Medicine (IOM) report focused on the physiological, psychological, and psychosocial effects of deployment-related stress. Findings revealed "sufficient evidence" of a positive association between deployment to a war zone and a number of specific health outcomes in studies in which chance and bias, including confounding, could be ruled out with reasonable confidence. The outcomes included psychiatric disorders, including PTSD, other anxiety disorders and depression; alcohol abuse; accidental death in the years after deployment;

suicide in the early years after deployment; and heightened marital and family conflict, such as intimate-partner violence (IOM, 2008).

Thus, military personnel returning from deployment in Iraq and Afghanistan—a part of the TRICARE beneficiary population that may have high demand for services—may present with a complex array of mental health and substance-use problems and psychosocial difficulties. Because many syndromes involve symptoms that mirror other mental and physical health diagnoses, advanced skills in differential clinical diagnosis are required to work with this client population.

Box 2.1 contains a fictitious vignette[2] featuring a returning OIF veteran viewed in the context of his partnership, family, and social environment. The diagnosis and course of treatment presented are intended to highlight the complexity and acuteness of the physical, psychological, and psychosocial issues confronted by clinicians who deliver services through TRICARE. This case is delineated in greater detail in Appendix F.

## MENTAL HEALTH CONDITIONS IDENTIFIED FOR ATTENTION BY THE TRICARE MANAGEMENT ACTIVITY

The committee's statement of task—spelled out in Chapter 1—lists several health outcomes that were identified for special attention by the TRICARE Management Activity. The sections below provide background information on them and briefly summarize their signs and symptoms, incidence, and recognized treatments. They are intended to provide context for understanding issues related to the diagnosis of and treatment for disorders that may be found in the TRICARE beneficiary population. In reviewing this text, it is important to consider that these conditions can co-occur in a person and make treatment needs complex.

More complete descriptions of the diagnostic criteria and etiology of these conditions are contained in the *Diagnostic and Statistical Manual of Mental Disorders* (*DSM*). A table in Chapter 5 (Table 5.3) lists examples of evidence-based psychosocial interventions for many of these disorders.

---

[2]The case was adapted and expanded from a clinical vignette contained in Basham (2009).

**BOX 2.1**
**Case Vignette—Sergeant Arrozo**
*Kathryn Basham, PhD, LICSW (Member of the Committee)*

Sergeant Carlos Arrozo, a 30-year-old Army OIF veteran of Puerto Rican descent, returned home after a 12-month tour of duty with second- and third-degree burns to his arms and face and a broken pelvis as a result of an IED blast. After his homecoming, he reunited with his 29-year-old wife of 10 years and his three young children, all under the age of 10 years. Although the reunion brought great relief and pride to the family, within 6 weeks Sgt. Arrozo started to experience pervasive anxiety, insomnia, and nightmares. Flashbacks of horrific combat experiences of violent actions were often triggered by smells of burning rubber, sights of men and women cloaked in heavily layered garments, sounds of cars backfiring, and visions of a vast expanse of sand blowing on the beach. Such events stimulated an intense traumatic stress response that activated arousal that alternated with numbness and detachment; this was consistent with posttraumatic stress and/or PTSD. Sgt. Arrozo's affect was totally dysregulated. When his wife, Maria, and children experienced terror during these episodes, they would retreat to safety as quickly as possible by hiding in distant rooms throughout the house or garage. Fighting ensued between the marital partners, with Sgt. Arrozo yelling at his children when they failed to follow his directives quickly enough. He sought refuge by drinking eight beers four or five times each week with his buddies and did not view this level of alcohol intake as a problem.

His home environment was characterized by fear, uncertainty, and detachment combined with pervasive anxiety in everyone involved. After receiving a medical discharge based on his physical injuries, PTSD, and depression, Sgt. Arrozo felt plagued by the impending threat of divorce, joblessness, and obsessional thoughts related to his "accidental killing" of a young child during combat. Sadness and unrelenting guilt overwhelmed him as he battled traumatic grief and depression, and they reactivated unresolved mourning surrounding his mother's death from cancer when he was 8 years old. In his words, Sgt. Arrozo felt "tense,

*continued*

**BOX 2.1 Continued**

distractible, agitated, irritable, enraged and numb" most of the time. Those symptoms not only are compatible with a diagnosis of PTSD but suggested syndromes of depression, substance abuse, or TBI. For example, sleeping poorly and suffering nightmares and headaches and then grogginess in the morning may be related to PTSD, or they could be related to depression, substance abuse, or TBI. The differential diagnosis of Sgt. Arrozo's distress leads to a complex nexus of PTSD, depression, TBI, substance abuse, and family conflict.

When Sgt. Arrozo agreed to seek mental health assistance, his wife telephoned to get access to a mental health provider authorized by TRICARE. After receiving the name of a nonmedical licensed mental health clinician, Sgt. Arrozo was invited to attend an individual session to embark on an assessment. After a 1-hour meeting, a preliminary diagnosis of PTSD and depression was established on the basis of a patient self-report. To help Sgt. Arrozo to find rapid relief from his combat-related psychological injuries, the clinician referred him to a colleague for prolonged exposure therapy and recommended meeting for 1 hour each week to address his symptoms of depression. The latter treatment plan included psychoeducation related to PTSD and depression and the use of cognitive-behavioral skills to track his depressed mood through journaling. Sgt. Arrozo could not concentrate on his daily writing assignments and felt ashamed of his incapacity to improve. After 3 weeks of the combined treatment plan, flooding of emotions from the exposure therapy overwhelmed him, and he decompensated, reporting many suicidal thoughts. He terminated the therapy.

## Major Depressive Disorder

Major depressive episodes are characterized by symptoms (Table 2.1) that are persistent and interfere with a person's daily living, functioning, and interactions with others (NIMH, 2009b). The episodes are not the result of normal bereavement due, for example, to the death of a loved one. Major depressive disorder (also known as major depression) is diagnosed when a person experiences one or more major depressive episodes

Was Sgt. Arrozo a failure, or were there unintended iatrogenic effects that were based on the absence of a thorough biopsychosocial assessment and differential diagnosis? Did the clinician fail to attend to the totality of this veteran's struggles and to explore areas in his social context (a faith-based community or cultural traditions, for example)? Were Sgt. Arrozo's competences, resilience at work and school, and military leadership skills explored and affirmed? Apparently, his undiagnosed mild TBI interfered with his benefiting from a cognitive-behavioral method that requires reasonably sound functioning. Finally, the absence of attunement to the volatile relationship between the marital partners and between the parents and children set the stage for increasing decompensation and further destabilization. Was a risk assessment completed to determine the safety or lack of safety in this home? Are there aspects of intimate-partner violence that are concealed? Are the children expressing symptoms of secondary trauma evidenced by heightened insecurity?

The treatment provided to Sgt. Arrozo and his family revealed various problems. They included an incomplete biopsychosocial assessment, inattention to safety risks, an inadequate treatment plan, the absence of collaboration with other providers, and lack of attunement to sociocultural influences. The complexity of the issues facing Sgt. Arrozo and his family requires strong clinical expertise that would permit a complex and detailed biopsychosocial assessment, including structured clinical interviews; the use of standardized clinical measures; and collaboration with other health professionals followed by a phase-oriented, relational, culturally responsive, and evidence-based practice plan.

A complete case summary of Sgt. Arrozo and his family is available in Appendix F.

with no history of manic symptoms. It is often an episodic illness, but persons with major depression can also experience chronic depressive symptoms (Judd et al., 1998).

The lifetime prevalence of major depression in the United States is nearly 17% (Kessler et al., 2005). In a study by Lapierre et al. (2007) of Iraq and Afghanistan war veterans, 37 and 38%, respectively, reported symptoms of depression. Hoge et al. (2004) found that 7.1–7.9% of troops returning from Iraq met criteria for depression and were

**TABLE 2.1** Criteria for Diagnosing Major Depressive Episodes

1. At least one of the following for at least 2 weeks:
   a. Depressed mood
   b. Markedly diminished interest or pleasure in all or almost all activities
2. And four or more of the following for at least 2 weeks:
   a. More than a 5% weight gain or loss, or increase or decrease in appetite
   b. Insomnia or hypersomnia
   c. Psychomotor agitation or retardation
   d. Fatigue or loss of energy
   e. Feelings of worthlessness or inappropriate guilt
   f. Indecisiveness or diminished concentration

NOTE: A diagnosis of major depression requires fulfillment of criteria beyond experiencing one or more major depressive episodes.
SOURCE: Adapted and abbreviated from APA (2000).

functionally impaired because of depressive symptoms, compared with 5.3% of troops who were about to be deployed.[3] Compounding the problem of depression in military veterans is the high prevalence of PTSD in this population. Campbell et al. (2007) report a study in which 36% of depressed patients in 10 VA primary-care practices screened positive for PTSD; these patients experienced more severe depressive symptoms, reported greater levels of anxiety and suicidal ideation, and were more likely to suffer a panic attack than patients who had depression without PTSD.

Because more soldiers now survive blasts that would previously have been fatal, TBI has become a serious concern for the military (Warden, 2006). Depression has been reported to follow TBI in 10–77% of cases (Alderfer et al., 2005).

The psychological effects of war are not limited to veterans themselves. Partners of veterans who have chronic PTSD have reported high levels of depression symptoms; 15% indicated recent suicidal ideation in one small study (Manguno-Mire et al., 2007).

---

[3]The unit surveyed before deployment was an Army unit. Two units returning from Iraq, one Army unit and one Marine Corps unit, were surveyed. The Marine Corps unit reported a 7.1% rate of depression, not statistically significantly different from the predeployment Army unit. The returning Army unit's depression rate was a statistically significantly different 7.9%. The "strict" criteria of depression required survey participants to indicate whether functioning at work, at home, or interpersonally was "very difficult." Rates of depression based on "broad" criteria are also reported in the study; these criteria leave out the requirement of functional impairment.

The VA/DOD (2009b) clinical practice guideline for major depressive disorder notes that co-occurring bipolar disorder, PTSD, substance-use disorder (SUD), suicidality/homicidality, and psychosis may complicate treatment or put the patient at increased risk for adverse outcomes. It also lists a number of pathobiologies associated with depression, including cardiovascular diseases, chronic pain syndromes, degenerative diseases, immune disorders, metabolic and endocrine conditions, neoplasms, and traumas such as TBI, amputation, and burn injuries. The guideline indicates that "[s]imultaneous treatment is often required for both the medical problem and psychiatric symptoms and can lead to overall improvement in function."

### Schizophrenia

Schizophrenia is a chronic illness in which patients experience episodes of psychosis (delusions or hallucinations) or disordered thought processes (Table 2.2). They often experience chronic negative symptoms characterized by a "flattening" of normal emotions or behavior. For example, a patient may exhibit an abnormally flat affect by speaking in a monotone or making few facial expressions. A person with schizophrenia may also demonstrate avolition, an inability to initiate and complete tasks, or alogia, a paucity of speech (APA, 2000; Moore and Jefferson, 2004e).

**TABLE 2.2** Summary of Major Diagnostic Criteria for Schizophrenia[a]

1. At least two of the following for a substantial portion of a 1-month period:
   a. Delusions
   b. Hallucinations
   c. Disorganized speech
   d. Grossly disorganized or catatonic behavior
   e. Negative symptoms, such as flattening of affect or avolition
2. Social or occupational dysfunction:
   a. Includes the 1 month of positive symptoms
   b. Other time may be occupied by negative symptoms
3. Overall duration of at least 6 months
4. Exclusion of schizoaffective and mood disorders
5. Exclusion of substance abuse or general medical conditions

[a]There are further criteria for the different subtypes.
SOURCE: Adapted and abbreviated from APA (2000).

The lifetime prevalence of schizophrenia in the general population is estimated at 0.2% (Kendler et al., 1996). The epidemiology of schizophrenia is different, however, in the military because current or past psychotic disorders disqualify applicants (NRC, 2006). In service members who develop schizophrenia, the average age at onset is later than that in the general population (Niebuhr et al., 2008).

## Posttraumatic Stress Disorder

Many people who have experienced a catastrophic event involving possible or actual injury, destruction, or death can be distressed, be fearful, or feel helpless. However, most people will recover from the experience. In cases of PTSD, recovery is incomplete. Patients exhibit symptoms that fall into three general categories: re-experiencing, avoidance, and hyperarousal (Table 2.3). Flashbacks and vivid nightmares of the traumatic experience are classic examples of re-experiencing symptoms. Re-experiencing symptoms may also be accompanied by panic attacks. Avoidance symptoms are characterized by the patient's taking steps to avoid stimuli that remind him or her of the original trauma. The stimuli might include conversations about the trauma and particular activities or locations. Examples of hyperarousal symptoms are difficulty in sleeping, irritability, and being easily startled. The *Diagnostic and Statistical Manual of Mental Disorders, Fourth Edition, Text Revision* (*DSM-IV-TR*) code for PTSD is 309.81 (APA, 2000).

In the general population, the lifetime prevalence of PTSD is nearly 7% (Kessler et al., 2005). Hoge et al. (2004) found symptoms of PTSD

**TABLE 2.3** General Diagnostic Criteria for PTSD[a]

1. The person experienced, directly or indirectly, a traumatic event; the person's response included intense fear, helplessness, or horror
2. One or more re-experience symptoms
3. Three or more avoidance symptoms
4. Two or more hyperarousal symptoms
5. Re-experience, avoidance, and hyperarousal symptoms last more than 1 month
6. Clinically significant distress or impairment results from the symptoms

[a]*DSM-IV-TR* contains more specific examples of re-experience, avoidance, and hyperarousal symptoms.
SOURCE: Adapted and abbreviated from APA (2000).

in 18% and 19.9% of survey respondents in two combat units returning from Iraq; members of the two units were over twice as likely to meet criteria for PTSD and to be functionally impaired by the symptoms as were survey participants in a predeployment unit (12.9% and 12.2% versus 5%). Co-occurrence of major depression and PTSD is common and requires more complex treatment (Campbell et al., 2007). A service member's PTSD can affect home and family dynamics; evidence suggests that the angry outbursts and emotional withdrawal associated with PTSD are the most damaging to family relationships (Galovski and Lyons, 2004). Family members are also at risk for PTSD themselves even though they did not directly experience the traumatic events. There have been cases in which children experienced many of the same PTSD symptoms as their Vietnam-veteran parents (Rosenheck and Nathan, 1985). In a small study of female spouses of returning Utah Army National Guard troops, 10.4% met the diagnostic criteria for PTSD (Renshaw et al., 2008).

There is abundant scientific evidence that PTSD can develop at any time after exposure to a traumatic stressor, including cases in which there is a long interval between the stressor and the recognition of symptoms. Some of the cases involve the initial onset of symptoms after many years of symptom-free life; others involve the manifestation of florid symptoms in persons with previously undiagnosed subclinical or subsyndromal PTSD (IOM, 2007).

The overlap of TBI and PTSD symptoms makes it challenging to differentiate the two conditions. Both diseases can cause irritability, difficulty in sleeping, and impairment of concentration. In general, the distinction is made by observing other symptoms: TBI tends to cause headaches, balance and visual disturbances, and hearing loss, whereas PTSD symptoms generally are restricted to the three categories mentioned above. But mild TBI can be particularly difficult to distinguish from PTSD (Labutta, 2009).

VA/DOD's (2004) clinical practice guideline lists a number of potential differential diagnoses or comorbidities associated with PTSD including dementia, depression, substance abuse/withdrawal, bereavement, psychosis, bipolar disease, seizure disorder, thyroid disease, neoplasms, somatization disorder, anxiety disorder, toxicosis, rheumatoid-collagen vascular disease, hypoxia, sleep apnea, closed-head injury, congestive heart failure, and delirium. It recommends that the existence of co-occurring disorders be considered when deciding whether to treat a patient in a primary care versus a specialty mental health care setting.

## Bipolar Disorder

Persons with bipolar disorder experience increased mood symptoms that are characterized as manic, hypomanic, or mixed (Tables 2.4–2.6). Manic episodes can include psychotic symptoms, such as hallucinations or delusions. Persons with bipolar disorder typically also experience periods of significant depression (Goodwin and Jamison, 2007).

The lifetime prevalence of bipolar I and II disorder in the general population is estimated to be nearly 4% (Kessler et al., 2005). Current bipolar disorder disqualifies someone for enlistment in the US military (NRC, 2006), but it is important to remember that bipolar disorder, although often episodic, is a chronic condition that requires continuing maintenance treatment.

## Mental Disorders Due to a General Medical Condition

Some general medical conditions can cause psychiatric symptoms or conditions. All those conditions share three diagnostic criteria (Table 2.7), the most prominent of which is a physical examination, history, or laboratory evidence pointing to a physiological cause. Examples

**TABLE 2.4** Major Diagnostic Criteria for a Manic Episode

1. At least three of the following:
    a. Inflated self-esteem or grandiosity
    b. Decreased need for sleep
    c. Increased talkativeness
    d. Feeling of racing thoughts
    e. Distractibility
    f. Increase in goal-directed activity
    g. Excessive involvement in potentially harmful activities (such as risky sexual activity, shopping sprees)
2. Symptoms last at least 1 week
3. Mood disturbance causes impairment of personal or social functioning or requires hospitalization

SOURCE: Adapted and abbreviated from APA (2000).

**TABLE 2.5** Major Diagnostic Criteria for a Mixed Episode

1. Criteria for both manic and major depressive episodes, except the duration criterion, are met nearly every day for 1 week
2. Social and occupational disruption results from the symptoms

SOURCE: Adapted and abbreviated from APA (2000).

**TABLE 2.6** Major Diagnostic Criteria for a Hypomanic Episode

1. A period of at least 4 days during which the patient's mood is persistently elevated, expansive, or irritable
2. At least three of the symptoms of a manic episode (four if the mood is only irritable)
3. Mood must be clearly different from the person's nonsymptomatic state
4. Mood change is observable by others
5. Episode is *not* severe enough to require hospitalization or impair social or occupational function

SOURCE: Adapted and abbreviated from APA (2000).

**TABLE 2.7** Common Diagnostic Criteria for All Mental Disorders Due to a General Medical Condition

1. History, physical examination, or laboratory evidence suggests a physiological cause
2. Another mental disorder does not account for the symptoms better
3. Symptoms are not restricted to periods of delirium

SOURCE: Adapted and abbreviated from APA (2000).

of possible physiologic causes are vitamin $B_{12}$ deficiency, heavy-metal poisoning, multiple sclerosis, and AIDS (Moore and Jefferson, 2004d). Biological causes should be distinguished from emotional triggers (Moore and Jefferson, 2004f). A patient might, for example, experience major depression after a heart attack when young. Unless a physiological link can be established between the heart damage and the depression, major depression is the appropriate diagnosis.

Treatment for a mental disorder that results from a general medical condition rests on resolving the underlying physical problem. In some cases, such as in hypoglycemia that results in delirium, the mental symptoms are easily resolved. In others, such as a stroke, complete reversal of the symptoms may not be achieved (Moore and Jefferson, 2004b).

## Somatoform Disorders

Somatoform disorders are manifested by physical symptoms that cannot be explained by the presence of a general medical condition. The symptoms may occur in the absence of any medical condition, or they may be in excess of what an existing medical condition would be expected to cause. Diagnostic criteria for two somatoform disorders—somatization disorder and pain disorder—are listed in Tables 2.8 and 2.9. The major distinction between somatoform disorders and such other conditions as malingering or factitious disorder is that the physical symptoms are not voluntarily created by a patient with a somatoform disorder (APA, 2000; Jacobson, 2001).

Estimates of the prevalence of somatoform disorder in primary-care populations range from 16% to 30% (De Waal et al., 2004; Fink et al., 1999). McCarroll et al. (2002) demonstrated an increase in somatic symptoms in mortuary workers during the Persian Gulf War. The subjects who had close contact with dead bodies (either by handling or by proximity to large numbers of bodies) at the Dover mortuary reported approximately twofold increases in scores on the Brief Symptom Inventory self-assessment of somatic symptoms. In another study of combat deployment, troops who had combat experience reported more severe somatic symptoms than troops who lacked combat experience; this

**TABLE 2.8** Major Diagnostic Criteria for Somatization Disorder (*DSM-IV-TR* code 300.81)

1. History of persistent physical complaints beginning before the age of 30 years; They result in treatment or substantial functional impairment
2. All the following must have been met at any point during the illness:
   a. Four pain symptoms
   b. Two gastrointestinal symptoms (not pain-related)
   c. One sexual symptom (not pain-related)
   d. One pseudoneurological symptom (not pain-related)
3. Either of the following:
   a. The symptoms above occur in the absence of a general medical condition or substance-related cause
   b. The symptoms above are in excess of what history and physical and laboratory findings would suggest
4. Symptoms are not intentionally produced or feigned

SOURCE: Adapted and abbreviated from APA (2000).

**TABLE 2.9** Major Diagnostic Criteria for Pain Disorder (*DSM-IV-TR* code 307.80)

1. Pain severe enough to justify clinical attention is the focus of the clinical visit
2. Pain causes substantial impairment in daily functioning
3. Onset, severity, exacerbation, or maintenance of pain has a substantial psychological component
4. Symptoms are not intentionally produced or feigned
5. Mood, anxiety, or psychotic disorders do not account for the pain better, nor does the pain satisfy the criteria for dyspareunia

SOURCE: Adapted and abbreviated from APA (2000).

relationship held even though the rates of PTSD in the two groups did not differ (Killgore et al., 2006).

In the general population, PTSD has been linked with more severe abridged somatization, defined by researchers as the presence of at least four somatization symptoms in men or at least six in women. A trend toward linking PTSD with increased risk of abridged somatization was found, but it was not statistically significant (Andreski et al., 1998).

### Delirium Associated with Head Trauma

Delirium is a medical emergency in which an underlying physiological condition causes acute or subacute global changes in cognitive functioning (Table 2.10). Patients are confused and have difficulty in focusing. Sleep–wake cycles may be altered, and the patient might be agitated. A hallmark of delirium is that it can "wax and wane" (i.e., a person with delirium can appear confused one moment but cogent later). Possible causes of delirium include extreme hypoglycemia, syphilis, substance abuse or withdrawal, severe body-temperature disturbances (hypothermia or hyperthermia), and brain infarct (Smith and Seirafi, 2006). In contrast with psychiatric conditions that might have similar symptoms, physical examination, patient history, and laboratory findings are suggestive of a physiological disturbance.

Delirium is a possible sequela of TBI. Nakase-Thompson et al. (2004) examined 85 consecutive TBI survivors admitted to a neurorehabilitation hospital. Of those patients, 59 (69%) met the *DSM-IV-TR* criteria for delirium due to a general medical condition at the time of admission. Not surprisingly, patients who had delirium had worse

**TABLE 2.10** Major Diagnostic Criteria for Delirium

1. Disturbance in ability to focus and direct attention
2. Change in cognition or development of perceptual disturbance that is not part of dementia
3. Acute onset (hours to days) and fluctuation throughout the day
4. History or physical examination or laboratory findings suggest a disturbance due to
   a. A general medical condition (*DSM-IV-TR* 293.0)
   b. Substance intoxication (*DSM-IV-TR* 291.0 for alcohol, *DSM-IV-TR* 292.81 for others)
   c. Substance withdrawal (*DSM-IV-TR* 291.0 for alcohol, *DSM-IV-TR* 292.81 for others)

SOURCE: Adapted and abbreviated from APA (2000).

scores on the Cognitive Test for Delirium and the Delirium Rating Scale than nondelirious patients. Diagnoses of delirium corresponded with more severe brain injury as measured by the number of contusions on a computed-tomography image. The increased severity of the patients' injuries was borne out by their worse scores on the Galveston Orientation and Amnesia Test, which measures orientation and memory of events surrounding a TBI, and the Agitated Behavior Scale (ABS), which measures agitation and distractibility of TBI patients. However, when other symptoms of delirium were controlled for, the ABS results became statistically nonsignificant.

Resolution of delirium requires proper diagnosis and treatment of the underlying medical condition. For example, some prescription drugs can impair cognitive function, so attention should be paid to identifying and eliminating or reducing the dosages of these drugs (Rudolph and Marcantonio, 2007). Delirium also must be properly differentiated from psychiatric conditions, such as depression, mania, and schizophrenia (Smith and Seirafi, 2006).

About 10% of patients hospitalized in general medical wards have delirium, although this rate increases to 16–24% in patients over 70 years old. In neurology services, the delirium prevalence increases to 40% (Smith and Seirafi, 2006), which is not surprising given the variety of neurological causes of delirium. No studies of delirium rates in veteran or military populations were found.

## Dementia Associated with Head Trauma

It is common for the elderly to experience mild memory loss and to have difficulty in recalling memories while still being able to form new memories. As long as the memory loss does not interfere with daily living, it is considered a normal part of the aging process (Richardson, 2001). Patients with dementia exhibit both short-term and long-term memory impairments and deficiencies in judgment, abstract thinking, and problem-solving skills. Hallucinations and delusions may also be present (Moore and Jefferson, 2004c). Patients commonly experience anxiety as part of the condition. Caretakers can be affected by the patients' progressive loss of independence (Kraus et al., 2008). Like delirium and amnesia, dementia is probably best characterized as a collection of symptoms caused by an underlying disease. Table 2.11 lists some of the possible causes of dementia. The specific *DSM-IV-TR* code for dementia depends on the etiology of the condition (APA, 2000).

Dementia is generally a chronic condition, and symptoms may or may not remain stable. There is no known cure for dementia of the Alzheimer type, and the symptoms worsen with time. However, a brain injury that results in dementia may leave symptoms that are relatively unchanging (Moore and Jefferson, 2004c). In some cases (3–29%), dementia may be at least partially reversed—for example, if it is caused by a vitamin deficiency (Reichman and Cummings, 2007).

There is debate about the relationship between TBI and dementia. A report from the Rotterdam Study found no significant correlation between head trauma and the risk of dementia of the Alzheimer type or other dementia (Mehta et al., 1999). But a study (Plassman et al., 2000) of US military veterans who had a confirmed past diagnosis of head trauma found that moderate and severe head injuries led to a higher risk

**TABLE 2.11** Examples of Possible Causes of Dementia

1. Huntington's disease
2. Vascular dementias
3. Vitamin $B_{12}$ deficiency
4. Folic acid deficiency
5. Neurosyphilis
6. Subdural hematoma

SOURCE: Adapted and abbreviated from APA (2000).

of dementia of Alzheimer type than that in patients who had no history of head injury (odds ratio [OR], 1.04–5.17 for moderate injuries; OR, 1.77–11.47 for severe injuries). Similar results were found when dementia of all types was considered (OR, 1.24–4.58 for moderate injuries; OR, 2.09–9.63 for severe injuries). In neither case did mild head injury lead to significant increases in the risk of dementia of Alzheimer type or other dementia.

A strong relationship is seen between age and dementia prevalence. Harvey et al. (2003) found that, starting at the age of 35 years, dementia prevalence roughly doubles with every 5 additional years of age. Of people 45–65 years old, 0.07–0.12 % have dementia, according to various studies (Harvey et al., 2003; Sampson et al., 2004). Of people over 65 years old, 5–10% have dementia. The prevalence increases to at least 30% in people over 80 years old (Moore and Jefferson, 2004c).

### Amnestic Disorders Associated with Head Trauma

Amnesia can be anterograde, characterized by the inability to form new memories, or retrograde, characterized by the inability to recall memories (Table 2.12). It is typically caused by an underlying general medical condition or a substance-related condition that involves a disturbance of the central nervous system. The typical amnesic episode has both anterograde and retrograde features, and episodes may be transient or chronic.

The time course of amnesia depends on the underlying cause. For example, an alcohol-induced blackout would produce transient amnesia, whereas damage to the temporal lobes would be more likely to produce

**TABLE 2.12** Major Diagnostic Criteria for Amnesia Due to a General Medical Condition (*DSM-IV-TR* 294.0)

1. An impairment in the ability to form new memories or recall previously acquired information
2. Impairment results in substantial loss of social or work functioning
3. Memory loss is not better accounted for by delirium or dementia
4. History or physical examination or laboratory findings suggest a physiological link to a general medical condition

SOURCE: Adapted and abbreviated from APA (2000).

chronic amnesia. Treatment for amnesia focuses on resolving the underlying cause (APA, 2000; Moore and Jefferson, 2004a).

For a diagnosis of amnesia, the symptoms must not be better accounted for by delirium or dementia. Delirium, although it includes elements of forgetfulness, also includes such symptoms as confusion and difficulty in focusing. Similarly, dementia features not only memory problems but deficiencies of executive functioning, abstract thinking, and problem solving (APA, 2000).

It has been well reported in the literature that TBI often results in memory loss involving events shortly before and after the injury. However, in considering the amnestic effects of TBI, it is important not to overlook the possible presence of delirium. Stuss et al. (1999) have argued that posttraumatic amnesia is better characterized as a confused state with symptoms akin to delirium. In fact, a review of the relationship between memory and moderate to severe TBI suggests that the memory loss that follows such injuries does not strictly meet the definition of pure amnesia (Vakil, 2005).

## Substance-Use Disorders

In the *Diagnostic and Statistical Manual of Mental Disorders,* SUDs are defined as substance abuse and dependence. A diagnosis of substance abuse (Table 2.13) requires a pattern of substance use that impairs a person's ability to meet personal, work, or social obligations; creates the risk of physical harm; or causes repeated legal problems. In contrast, substance dependence (Table 2.14) is characterized by an increasing preoccupation with getting, using, or recovering from use of a substance

**TABLE 2.13** Major Diagnostic Criteria for Substance Abuse

1. A pattern of substance use characterized by one or more of the following in a 12-month period:
   a. Recurrent substance use leading to failure to fulfill major work, school, or home obligations
   b. Recurrent substance use in situations where it is physically hazardous
   c. Recurrent legal problems resulting from substance use
   d. Continued substance use despite recurring social disturbances resulting from it
2. Symptoms have never met criteria for substance dependence

SOURCE: Adapted and abbreviated from APA (2000).

**TABLE 2.14** Major Diagnostic Criteria for Substance Dependence

A pattern of substance use characterized by three or more of the following in a 12-month period:

1. Tolerance to the substance
2. Withdrawal signs
3. Substance is taken in larger quantities or for longer periods than intended
4. A persistent desire or unsuccessful efforts to reduce substance use
5. Much time is spent on efforts to obtain the substance or to recover from its effects
6. Substance use interferes with major social, occupational, or recreational activities
7. Substance use continues despite knowledge that it is causing or exacerbating a recurrent physical or psychological disturbance

SOURCE: Adapted and abbreviated from APA (2000).

to the extent that a person experiences impaired functioning and an inability to decrease or discontinue substance use. Tolerance (needing to take increasing amounts of a substance to become intoxicated or a failure of a given amount of the substance to create the same level of intoxication) and the occurrence of withdrawal symptoms on discontinuation of use of a substance can indicate dependence, but they are not necessary for the diagnosis (APA, 2000).

Persons with SUDs are at higher risk for a co-occurring mental illness. The reverse is also true: mental illness is a risk factor for SUD (Kessler, 2004). Patients who have co-occurring SUD and other psychiatric illnesses tend to have a more complicated and chronic course of illness (Greenfield et al., 1998; Kessler, 2004). Treating a person for a co-occurring psychiatric disorder (Cornelius et al., 1997; Greenfield et al., 1998) and remission of its symptoms (Hasin et al., 1996) can improve SUD outcomes. The VA/DOD (2009c) clinical practice guideline for management of SUDs recommends that the management of co-occurring medical and psychiatric conditions be prioritized and singles out cessation treatment for patients with nicotine dependence. The guideline also recommends that patients should be assessed for unmet psychosocial needs or situational stressors, including inadequate housing or homelessness, poor social supports, and problematic family relationships or situations.

The prevalence of SUDs in the general population is nearly 15% (Kessler et al., 2005). Research in military populations shows that combat deployment to Iraq and Afghanistan is associated with increased rates of alcohol misuse. Hoge et al. (2004) found that members of Army and Marine Corps units returning from deployment were more likely than members of units before deployment to use alcohol more than intended or to experience desires to reduce their drinking.[4] SUD has also been linked with PTSD in various studies of veterans' health. A study by Bremner et al. (1996) of Vietnam veterans found that as their PTSD symptoms worsened, so did their abuse of alcohol and other drugs. Patients who have PTSD experience more hospitalizations than patients who do not; this suggests that comorbid PTSD worsens outcomes of treatment for substance abuse (Brown et al., 1995). Support for that idea comes from Brown and Stout (1997), who reported that in patients who had both alcohol-use disorders and PTSD, remitted PTSD was associated with consumption of fewer drinks. However, they also reported that in patients who had active PTSD, remission of alcoholism was not associated with a difference in PTSD symptoms.

It is generally well recognized that SUD, with resulting motor and decision-making impairment during intoxication, is a risk factor for TBI (Graham and Cardon, 2008). However, relatively little research has been done on substance abuse following TBI. Horner et al. (2005) conducted a study to understand post-TBI alcohol consumption, a clinically relevant concern because excessive drinking after TBI can lead to seizures, further TBI, and less successful rehabilitation. Among their findings was that few patients increased their drinking 1 year after a TBI: 58% drank the same amount, and 36% drank less. Even among study participants who described themselves as moderate or heavy drinkers, almost half said that they drank less than before their TBI. Risk factors for increased alcohol consumption included depression after TBI and a pre-TBI history of substance abuse. TBI severity did not correlate with the quantity of alcohol consumed.

### Other Disorders Regularly Associated with Head Trauma

TBI and intracranial hemorrhage are commonly associated with head trauma and can result in behavioral changes or impairment of mental status. Their incidence is not mutually exclusive: hemorrhage

[4]In the control group of predeployment soldiers, 17.2% reported using alcohol more than intended, and 12.5% reported feeling the need to reduce alcohol consumption. In contrast, excess alcohol use was reported in 24.5%, 24.2%, and 35.4% of troops in two postdeployment Army units and one Marine Corps unit. Similarly, in the postdeployment units, 18.2%, 20.6%, and 29.4% reported feeling a need to reduce alcohol consumption.

can easily accompany a TBI. Epilepsy, through its association with severe TBI, is also linked to head trauma. TBI commonly accompanies skull fractures, although skull fracture itself does not necessarily lead to behavioral changes.

### *Traumatic Brain Injury*

TBI is typically described as mild, moderate, or severe; the distinctions vary among authors and organizations. Lowenstein (2009) identifies the criteria in Table 2.15 as commonly accepted for the three categories of TBI. Injuries may be open (e.g., from a missile wound to the head) or closed (e.g., from falling and striking the head). In the OIF and OEF conflicts in Iraq and Afghanistan, the classic cause of TBI is blast, which may lead to either open or closed injuries. From January 2003 to April 2006, 28% of the Iraq and Afghanistan combat casualties treated at Walter Reed Army Medical Center had a TBI (Labutta, 2009). One of the most prominent theories of the mechanism of blast-related closed-head injuries suggests that the overpressure and underpressure waves created by an explosion can damage the brain (Jaffee, 2009).

The symptoms of TBI include several that overlap with PTSD, including irritability, difficulty in concentrating, and insomnia. It can therefore be challenging, especially in mild cases of TBI, to differentiate it from PTSD. As a general principle, TBI includes additional physical symptoms, such as headache, vision and balance disturbances, and hearing loss. Such symptoms are not usually associated with PTSD (Labutta, 2009). VA/DOD (2009a) clinical practice guideline lists chronic pain, mood disorders, stress disorder, and personality disorder among the

**TABLE 2.15** Common Criteria for Judging the Severity of Traumatic Brain Injury

| Severity | Ctiteria |
|---|---|
| Mild | Loss of consciousness for under 30 minutes without skull fracture |
| Moderate | Loss of consciousness for over 30 minutes and under 24 hours with or without skull fracture |
| Severe | Loss of consciousness for over 24 hours with contusion, hematoma, or skull fracture |

SOURCE: Lowenstein (2009).

common co-occurring conditions for mild TBI. It also notes that SUDs may exacerbate or maintain the presentation of mild TBI symptoms and must be screened for.

### *Epilepsy Following Traumatic Brain Injury*

Epileptic seizures are alterations in behavior caused by hyperactive neural discharges in the brain. They are time-limited and occur suddenly. The signs and symptoms depend on the kind of seizure. Although the stereotypical seizures involve losing consciousness, collapsing to the ground, and convulsing (generalized tonic–clonic seizures), other seizures might appear as brief inattentiveness (absence seizures) or cause symptoms localized to specific organ systems or regions (partial seizures) (Spencer, 2007). Epileptic seizures can be due to disturbances intrinsic to the brain itself, or they can be provoked by extrinsic factors, such as a fever. Some 10% of people who reach the age of 70 years will have experienced an epileptic seizure. A single epileptic seizure, however, is not generally sufficient to justify a diagnosis of epilepsy. A formal diagnosis of epilepsy requires the occurrence of repeated, unprovoked seizures. Medication can be helpful in reducing the incidence of epileptic seizures (St. Louis and Granner, 2008).

Seizures are not uncommon after a TBI, although, as in the general population, the diagnosis of epilepsy requires recurrent seizures. One approach to characterizing seizures after TBI is to group them temporally. Immediate seizures occur less than 24 hours after the injury, early seizures occur within a week, and late seizures occur more than a week after the injury; it is the occurrence of multiple late seizures that warrants a diagnosis of epilepsy (Lowenstein, 2009). The risk of experiencing an unprovoked seizure is tied to the severity of the TBI. One study reported that the relative risk, compared with that in the general population, of a seizure was 1.5 (95% confidence interval [CI], 1.0–2.2) in patients with mild TBI, 2.9 (95% CI, 1.9–4.1) in patients with moderate TBI, and 17 (95% CI, 12.3–23.6) in patients with severe TBI. Furthermore, in patients with severe TBI, the risk of a first-time unprovoked seizure remained increased for over 10 years after the injury (Annegers et al., 1998). Given the high incidence of severe TBI in returning Iraq and Afghanistan veterans, this population is probably at much higher risk of epilepsy in the years to come.

### *Intracranial Hemorrhage*

There are four types of intracranial hemorrhage, each of which presents in a different manner. As blood leaks from damaged vessels, it forms a hematoma and can clot. Death may result from uncontrolled bleeding or from a clot that becomes too large. An epidural hematoma typically occurs when an artery is damaged and allows blood to leak into the space between the dura mater (the outermost of three membranes surrounding the brain) and the inside of the skull. The brain itself is not usually injured. Symptoms, including loss of consciousness, are typically observed within 2 hours of the initial injury.

Subdural hematomas classically result from leakage of blood from a vein underneath the dura mater. Direct damage to the brain is a common feature. When a subdural hematoma is present with a TBI, the patient is at increased risk for epilepsy (Annegers et al., 1998). Subdural hematomas can also develop insidiously from slow bleeding; in such cases, subtle physical and mental symptoms resulting from the hematoma's presence may develop over the course of days and may be difficult to notice. Intracranial hemorrhage is the loss of blood directly into the brain and can result in extremely rapid death. Finally, subarachnoid hemorrhage usually results from leakage from small blood vessels into the cerebrospinal fluid that fills the space between the surface of the brain and the arachnoid mater (the innermost membrane surrounding the brain) (Cantu, 2003).

### *Co-occurring (Polytrauma) Disorders*

VA defines polytrauma as "two or more injuries to physical regions or organ systems, one of which may be life threatening, resulting in physical, cognitive, psychological, or psychosocial impairments and functional disability" (Department of Veterans Affairs, 2009). TBI due to blast may be the signature injury in veterans of the wars in Iraq and Afghanistan. Explosions, by their nature, are likely to damage several regions or functional systems of the body and therefore are major causes of polytrauma in the military. In contrast, the most common cause of polytrauma in a civilian setting is automobile accidents (Friedemann-Sánchez et al., 2008).

A chart review (Sayer et al., 2008) of 188 patients admitted to the four VA polytrauma rehabilitation centers (PRCs) found that polytrauma patients injured by blast were more disabled than polytrauma patients whose injuries were caused by other means. Blast survivors had a greater number of total injuries to their bodies, were more likely to have suffered limb amputation, and had more skin and soft-tissue burns or wounds. They were also more likely than nonblast-polytrauma patients to experience PTSD symptoms (42% versus 24%). Rates of depressive, non-PTSD anxiety, and psychotic symptoms did not differ between the two groups.

The complicated nature of polytrauma patients makes it difficult to create effective treatment plans for them. One PRC staff member recounted, in an interview with researchers (Friedemann-Sánchez et al., 2008), a patient who had attention and memory deficits with PTSD. Ordinarily, the staff member would treat the attention and memory deficits with a stimulant medication, but the PTSD and associated agitation and anxiety made this approach unworkable. Another staff member quoted by the researchers noted that pain can be an important barrier to effective treatment, saying "when you have such tremendous pain you can't concentrate. How do you put cognition in front of somebody who is in excruciating pain? Then you give them medication, they don't hurt, but they can't think."

To care more effectively for service members who have experienced polytrauma, VA established the Polytrauma System of Care (PSC). It consists of four PRCs to handle acute rehabilitation, 21 polytrauma network sites to provide postacute inpatient and outpatient rehabilitation, and teams of polytrauma specialists at over 70 smaller VA facilities. Contact people are available at VA facilities that lack specialized polytrauma support. The PSC also includes a telehealth network to help to provide follow-up care to veterans in rural or underserved areas and in-theater consultations (Jaffee, 2009). Rehabilitation is an interdisciplinary process, involving specialists in physical medicine and rehabilitation, nursing, social work, physical therapy, rehabilitation psychology, and other fields. Because rehabilitation takes an emotional toll on both patients and families, the interdisciplinary teams consider the needs not only of the patients but of family members (Collins and Kennedy, 2008).

## PSYCHOSOCIAL ISSUES IN US MILITARY FAMILIES

In addition to the disorders discussed above, TRICARE beneficiaries are at special risk for some psychosocial problems. These problems are addressed below.

### Increased Marital Conflict

Multiple deployments and longer deployments are directly associated with increased mental health problems in service members and increased marital conflict (MHAT, 2006). A 2008 IOM report contains a review of two primary and three secondary studies of Vietnam veterans who had combat-related PTSD; they showed a direct association between combat exposure and an increase in marital conflict that persisted for many years after the war (IOM, 2008). Studies have reported that service members often return with heightened tendencies toward interpersonal conflicts and more interpersonal aggressive ideation, characteristics that increase the potential for marital conflict (Milliken et al., 2009).

### Increased Divorce Rates

Couples that experience increased marital and family conflict at any phase of the deployment cycle often move toward separation and divorce. The decision to divorce commonly comes while the service member is deployed, and this adds to the marital and family conflict and the potential for mental health distress. Not only are both partners affected by the stress of marital dissolution but children and extended family are distressed. Families may experience financial difficulties and estrangement from friends and family, which may contribute to adverse effects on mental health.

### Increased Intimate-Partner Violence

The literature on the effects of deployment on the perpetration of intimate-partner violence (IPV) by veterans against spouses and partners is extensive. One large primary study conducted in the early 1990s revealed an association between deployment and increased IPV perpetrated by active-duty soldiers (Jordan et al., 1992), and aggression increased with the length of deployment. Campbell and colleagues (2003) report a lifetime IPV prevalence of 30% in a sample of 616 active-duty military women; the prevalence during military service was 21.6%. Three other studies that used data from the National Vietnam Veterans Readjustment Survey (NVVRS) on spouses and partners of Vietnam veterans found an association between combat-related PTSD and increased IPV. A more recent study conducted by Fonseca et al. (2006) confirmed that lower age, more stress, and alcohol use are important individual predictors, in addition to combat exposure, of IPV. Other studies focused on an association of deployment and an increased incidence of interpersonal violence outside the family.

Recent studies suggest that male service members and unemployed male spouses of service members are also victims of IPV, indicating that male victims suffer long-term effects similar to those in females but may be reluctant to seek care (Bell, 2009; Newby et al., 2003). When there are power shifts or status inconsistencies in the marital relationships, there is an increased risk of IPV.

Newspaper and magazine articles have reported an increase in intimate-partner femicide, the most severe form of IPV, among male service members who returned from Iraq and Afghanistan (Alvarez, 2008; Alvarez and Sontag, 2008). It is speculated that depression, PTSD, and the focus on military combat behaviors—as well as access to weapons—is related to the increased femicide of spouses. Many women are reluctant to disclose IPV because of the military's mandatory reporting policy, loss of confidentiality, and fear of an effect of reporting on the careers of the service members and on their families. For that reason, routine screening of all women for IPV is thought to be important for the military health-care setting. Screening may increase referrals to other services, such as those for alcohol or drug treatment, and parenting classes that might reduce or prevent further victimization and its consequences (Chapin and Mackie, 2007).

A 2008 IOM report concluded that there is "sufficient evidence" of an association between deployment to a war zone and later marital and family conflict, including IPV. The association is especially strong when a service member has a diagnosis of PTSD. Not only is combat exposure associated with increased IPV, but soldiers and marines who had mental health problems were more likely to mistreat noncombatants, demonstrating heightened aggression. A meta-analysis of 64 published reports in 2005 revealed increased rates of IPV in military populations. For both military veterans and active-duty service members, IPV results in substantial victim injury (Marshall et al., 2005). Interventions for IPV include the so-called *Duluth model*—a treatment that focuses on power and control issues—and cognitive-behavior treatment. However, empirical support for their efficacy is lacking (Stover et al., 2009).

## Suicide

In recent years, suicide rates among warfighters and veterans have increased, raising concerns among mental health professionals who need to determine the most effective prevention and clinical practice models to help patients struggling with suicidal ideation and behavior. Suicide rates among service members have spiked since 2001, coincident with the initiation of Operation Iraqi Freedom operations. Army data released in December 2009 indicate that rates rose every year between 2005 and 2009 (DOD, 2009a). The 2008 *Department of Defense Survey of Health-Related Behaviors Among Active-Duty Military Personnel* reported attempted suicide rates of 2.8% in the US Navy, 2.3% in the Marines, 2.0% in the Army, 1.7% in the Coast Guard, and 1.6% in the Air Force (DOD, 2009b). These represent a doubling of the rates observed in 2005. Accurate accounting is difficult, though, because of the reluctance to report suicidal ideation and gestures, and the fact that some deaths reported as accidents involve suicidal intent.

In response to these events, the US Army and the National Institute of Mental Health initiated the Army Study to Assess Risk and Resilience in Servicemembers in 2008. This study, the largest of suicide and mental health among military personnel ever undertaken, is intended to identify risk and protective factors to help the Army develop effective strategies for mitigating suicide risk (NIMH, 2009a).

## Mental Health Issues in Children

A landmark study codirected by Rosenheck and Fontana (1998) analyzed NVVRS data on family violence, child behavior, and family cohesion and found that behavior problems in the children of veterans were associated with their veteran parents' participation in abusive violence. It also reported more depression in children of deployed veterans. Intergenerational transmission of trauma was demonstrated: abusive violence during the Vietnam era was associated with behavioral and mental health disturbances in the veterans' children 10–15 years later. A study by Samper et al. (2004) explored relationships between PTSD and parenting satisfaction. Findings suggest that higher levels of PTSD symptoms, particularly numbness and avoidance, may have a deleterious effect on parent–child relationships. A primary study by Jensen et al. (1996) found that children who had one parent deployed to the Gulf War had more behavioral dysfunction; boys were at greater risk than girls for depression associated with the parent's deployment.

A cross-sectional study of 169 consenting families aimed at describing the effect of wartime military deployments on the behavior of young children in military families found that children who were at least 3 years old and had a deployed parent exhibited more behavioral symptoms than their peers who did not have a deployed parent when caregivers' stress and depressive symptoms were controlled for (Chartrand et al., 2008). In a study of the effects of deployment on the maltreatment of children, Rentz et al. (2007) conducted a time-series analysis of Texas child-maltreatment data for 2000–2003 to examine changes in the occurrence of child maltreatment in military and nonmilitary families. The rate of substantiated child maltreatment in military families was twice as high in the period after October 2002 as before. Nonmilitary caretakers perpetrated the largest proportion of maltreatment of children, and this suggests that the transitions and separations related to deployment imposed great stressors on the families. In FY 1998–2007, cases of child abuse reported to the DOD Family Advocacy Program (2008) varied from 11.4 to 14.9 per 1,000 children; the substantiated rate of abuse was 4.9–7.3 per 1,000.[5]

## Incarceration

An IOM committee (2008) concluded that there was limited but suggestive evidence of an association between deployment and incarceration. Recent studies have pointed to the distinctly higher rates of suicide in incarcerated veterans than in nonveteran prisoners. A veteran in jail has a suicide risk beyond that conferred by either veteran status or incarceration alone (Wortzel et al., 2009). There is clearly a need to offer specialized assessment and clinical practice interventions in the incarcerated veteran population.

[5]DOD cautioned against comparing these data with data from other studies unless differences in contexts, methods, data elements, and demographics were standardized for military populations.

### Employment, Finances, and Homelessness

A previous IOM (2008) research effort concluded that there was inadequate evidence to determine whether an association exists between deployment and homelessness and adverse employment outcomes. That conclusion may have been driven by the dearth of methodologically rigorous studies available at the time. More recent anecdotal reports of the transitions of OEF and OIF veterans suggest increasing difficulty with financial stability, employment, and housing (MHAT, 2006). Because social supports remain the major protective factors in mediating adverse mental health outcomes while also promoting healing, attention should be focused on the social contexts of service members and their families during any phase of clinical intervention.

## DATA ON PATIENTS UNDER THE CARE OF COUNSELORS

In the statement of task, TRICARE requested that the committee review and synthesize available data on the proportions of all patients who had a series of specified disorders and were under the care of licensed mental health counselors. The committee requested those data from the TRICARE Management Activity; the information listed in Table 2.16 is derived from its response to the request. It is important to note several limitations of the information. The table provides estimates of the numbers of cases treated in the TRICARE population, but for several reasons it probably does not reflect the true prevalences of the disorders. The gold standard for determining diagnoses is the structured clinical interview or chart review. The information in Table 2.16 was obtained from administrative data based on usual care practice, which often does not include structured diagnostic interviews by clinicians and therefore can be less accurate. Research shows that accuracy of claims data can vary by diagnosis. For example, administrative data have demonstrated relatively high accuracy for bipolar disorder (Unutzer et al., 1998, 2000) and schizophrenia (Lurie et al., 1992) but lower accuracy for depression (Spettel et al., 2003). In addition, this information reflects only the primary (or first) diagnosis entered in an insurance claim; if a patient presented for treatment and the mental and substance-use (M/SU) condition was not listed first (e.g., depression and SUD or hypertension and generalized anxiety), the condition would not be included in the table. Therefore, the table likely underrepresents the prevalence of these

**TABLE 2.16** Patients in the Care of Mental Health Counselors in the Military Health System

| | TRICARE Beneficiaries with Diagnosis During FY 2008 | | |
|---|---|---|---|
| Diagnosis | Total (*N*) | Seen by Mental Health Counselor[a] (*N*) | Seen by Mental Health Counselor (% of enrollees with M/SU diagnosis) |
| Major depressive disorder | 204,078 | 10,480 | 5.1 |
| Schizophrenia | 4,335 | 182 | 4.2 |
| Posttraumatic stress disorder | 36,526 | 2,484 | 6.8 |
| Bipolar disorder | 40,970 | 2,573 | 6.3 |
| Mental health disorder related to a general medical condition | 9,681 | 144 | 1.5 |
| Somatoform disorder | 529 | 9 | 1.7 |
| Delirium | 586 | 1 | 0.2 |
| Dementia | 1,042 | 8 | 0.8 |
| Amnestic disorder | 188 | 3 | 1.6 |
| Substance-use disorder | 66,067 | 974 | 1.1 |
| Traumatic brain injury | 38,159 | 11 | 0.03 |

[a]Data may include providers who have different levels of licensure, certification, education, and experience.
SOURCE: TMA (2009).

disorders in the treatment-seeking TRICARE population. Finally, the table does not capture the complexity of co-occurring medical, M/SU, and psychosocial problems that are often seen in this population.

Information provided to the committee indicates there were 9,197,927 TRICARE beneficiaries in FY 2008 (TMA, 2009). However, the data in Table 2.16 excludes TRICARE for Life participants because TRICARE is not their primary payer. Enrollees in the six designated provider plans are also excluded. This reduces the overall number of beneficiaries for whom outcomes are reported in the table to 7,217,566.

The committee attempted to identify and obtain other available data on the proportions of patients who had various diagnoses and were under the care of licensed mental health counselors. However, such data are not present in the scientific literature and are not routinely compiled by care providers.[6] Even if they were, the weaknesses in the TRICARE data identified above suggest that they would be of little utility in evaluating the ability of counselors to provide services to the TRICARE beneficiary population as independent practitioners.

## REFERENCES

Alderfer BS, Arciniegas DB, Silver JM. 2005. Treatment of depression following traumatic brain injury. *Journal of Head Trauma Rehabilitation* 20(6):544-562.

Alvarez L. 2008. Despite Army assurances: Violence at home. *New York Times*, November 23, 2008, 24.

Andreski P, Chilcoat H, Breslau N. 1998. Post-traumatic stress disorder and somatization symptoms: A prospective study. *Psychiatry Research* 79(2):131-138.

Annegers JF, Hauser WA, Coan SP, Rocca WA. 1998. A population-based study of seizures after traumatic brain injuries. *New England Journal of Medicine* 338(1):20-24.

APA (American Psychiatric Association). 2000. *Diagnostic and statistical manual of mental disorders,* 4th ed., text revision. Washington, DC: American Psychiatric Association.

Basham K. 2009. "Commentary on the keynote lecture presented by Dr. Jonathan Shay, Friday, June 27, 2008, titled 'The trials of homecoming: Odysseus returns from Iraq/Afghanistan, and additional reflections.'" *Smith College Studies in Social Work* 79(3&4):299-309.

Bell N. 2009. Health and occupational consequences of spouse abuse victimization among male U.S. Army soldiers. *Journal of Interpersonal Violence* 24(5):751-769.

Bremner JD, Southwick SM, Darnell A, Charney DS. 1996. Chronic PTSD in Vietnam combat veterans: Course of illness and substance abuse. *American Journal of Psychiatry* 153(3):369-375.

Brown PJ, Stout RL. 1997. *Six-month posttreatment outcomes of substance use disordered patients with and without comorbid PTSD.* Paper presented at the annual meeting of the International Society for Traumatic Stress Studies, Montreal, Ontario, Canada.

Brown PJ, Recupero PR, Stout R. 1995. PTSD substance abuse comorbidity and treatment utilization. *Addictive Behavior* 20(2):251-254.

Campbell DG, Felker BL, Liu CF, Yano EM, Kirchner JE, Chan D, Rubenstein LV, Chaney EF. 2007. Prevalence of depression-PTSD comorbidity: Implications for clinical practice guidelines and primary care-based interventions. *Journal of General Internal Medicine* 22(6):711-718.

Campbell JC, Garza MA, Gielen AC, O'Campo P, Kub J, Dienemann J, Jones AS, Jafar E. 2003. Intimate partner violence and abuse among active duty military women. *Violence Against Women* 9(9):1072-1092.

---

[6]Some researchers have examined the proportion of patients in the general population (Wang et al., 2005, 2006) or particular demographic groups (Neighbors et al., 2006) under the care of psychiatrists versus nonpsychiatrists, but these publications do not differentiate counselors from other nonpsychiatrist providers.

Cantu RC. 2003. Head injuries. In *Delee and Drez's orthopaedic sports medicine,* 2nd ed., edited by DeLee JC, Drez DJ, Miller MD. Philadelphia: Saunders Elsevier.

Chapin MG, Mackie CF. 2007. Research evidence to update practice guidelines for domestic violence screening in military settings. *Military Medicine* 172(7):ii-iv.

Chartrand MM, Frank DA, White LF, Shope TR. 2008. Effect of parents' wartime deployment on the behavior of young children in military families. *Archives of Pediatrics and Adolescent Medicine* 162(11):1009-1014.

Collins RC, Kennedy MC. 2008. Serving families who have served: Providing family therapy and support in interdisciplinary polytrauma rehabilitation. *Journal of Clinical Psychology* 64(8):993-1003.

Cornelius JR, Salloum IM, Ehler JG, Jarrett PJ, Cornelius MD, Perel JM, Thase ME, Black A. 1997. Fluoxetine in depressed alcoholics: A double-blind, placebo-controlled trial. *Archives of General Psychiatry* 54(8):700-705.

Cully JA, Zimmer M, Khan MM, Petersen LA. 2008. Quality of depression care and its impact on health service use and mortality among veterans. *Psychiatric Services* 59(12):1399-1405.

de Waal MW, Arnold IA, Eekhof JA, van Hemert AM. 2004. Somatoform disorders in general practice: Prevalence, functional impairment and comorbidity with anxiety and depressive disorders. *British Journal of Psychiatry* 184(6):470-476.

Department of Veterans Affairs. 2009. *Definitions—VA polytrauma system of care.* http://www.polytrauma.va.gov/definitions.asp#polytrauma. (Accessed July 16, 2009).

DOD (Department of Defense). 2007a. *Demographics 2007: Profile of the military community.* http://cs.mhf.dod.mil/content/dav/mhf/QOL-Library/Project%20Documents/MilitaryHOMEFRONT/Reports/2007%20Demographics.pdf. (Accessed July 28, 2009).

DOD. 2007b. *An achievable vision: Report of the Department of Defense Task Force on Mental Health.* Falls Church, VA: Defense Health Board.

DOD. 2009a. *Army suicide rate increases five straight years.* American Forces Press Service release, December 11. http://www.defense.gov/news/newsarticle.aspx?id=57086. (Accessed January 1, 2010).

DOD. 2009b. *2008 Department of Defense survey of health related behaviors among active duty military personnel. A component of the Defense lifestyle assessment program (DLAP).* Prepared by RTI International, September. http://www.tricare.mil/2008HealthBehaviors.pdf. (Accessed January 1, 2010).

DOD Family Advocacy Program. 2008. *Child Abuse and Domestic Abuse Data Trends from FY 1998 to 2007.* Information Paper. http://cs.mhf.dod.mil/content/dav/mhf/QOL-Library/Project%20Documents/MilitaryHOMEFRONT/Homepage/CADA%20trends98-07%20no%20contact%20info.pdf. (Accessed November 7, 2009).

Donohoe M. 2005. Violence against women in the military. *Medscape Ob/Gyn & Women's Health* 10(2). http://www.medscape.com/viewarticle/512380. (Accessed January 8, 2010).

Eaton KM, Hoge CW, Messer SC, Whitt AA, Cabrera MS, McGurk D, Cox A, Castro CA. 2008. Prevalence of mental health problems, treatment, need, and barriers to care among primary care-seeking spouses of military service members involved in Iraq and Afghanistan deployments. *Military Medicine* 173(11):1051-1056.

Fink P, Sørensen L, Engberg M, Holm M, Munk-Jørgensen P. 1999. Somatization in primary care: Prevalence, health care utilization, and general practitioner recognition. *Psychosomatics* 40(4):330-338.

Fonseca CA, Schmaling KB, Stoever C, Gutierrez C, Blume AW, Russell ML. 2006. Variables associated with intimate partner violence in a deploying military sample. *Military Medicine* 171(7):627-631.

Friedemann-Sánchez G, Sayer NA, Pickett T. 2008. Provider perspectives on rehabilitation of patients with polytrauma. *Archives of Physical Medicine and Rehabilitation* 89(1):171-178.

Friedman MJ. 2006. Posttraumatic stress disorder among military returnees from Afghanistan and Iraq. *American Journal of Psychiatry* 163(4):586-593.

Galovski T, Lyons JA. 2004. Psychological sequelae of combat violence: A review of the impact of PTSD on the veteran's family and possible interventions. *Aggression and Violent Behavior* 9(5):477-501.

Goldzweig CL, Balekian TM, Rolon C, Yano EM, Shekelle PG. 2006. The state of women veterans' health research: Results of a systematic literature review. *Journal of General Internal Medicine* 21(Suppl. 3):S82-S92.

Goodwin FK, Jamison KR. 2007. Manic-depressive illness. New York: Oxford University Press.

Graham DP, Cardon AL. 2008. An update on substance use and treatment following traumatic brain injury. *Annals of the New York Academy of Sciences* 1141:148-162.

Greenfield SF, Weiss RD, Muenz LR, Vagge LM, Kelly JF, Bello LR, Michael J. 1998. The effect of depression on return to drinking: A prospective study. *Archives of General Psychiatry* 55(3):259-265.

Harvey RJ, Skelton-Robinson M, Rossor MN. 2003. The prevalence and causes of dementia in people under the age of 65 years. *Journal of Neurology, Neurosurgery & Psychiatry* 74(9):1206-1209.

Hasin DS, Tsai W-Y, Endicott J, Mueller TI, Coryell W, Keller M. 1996. The effects of major depression on alcoholism: Five-year course. *American Journal on Addictions* 5(2):144-155.

HealthNet Federal Services. 2009. *The TRICARE North region.* https://www.hnfs.net/common/companyInfo/TRICARE_North_Region_Health_Net.htm. (Accessed July 28, 2009).

Hoge CW, Castro CA, Messer SC, McGurk D, Cotting DI, Koffman RL. 2004. Combat duty in Iraq and Afghanistan, mental health problems, and barriers to care. *New England Journal of Medicine* 351(1):13-22.

Hoge CW, Terhakopian A, Castro CA, Messer SC, Engel CC. 2007. Association of posttraumatic stress disorder with somatic symptoms, health care visits, and absenteeism among Iraq war veterans. *American Journal of Psychiatry* 164(1):150-153.

Horner MD, Ferguson PL, Selassie AW, Labbate LA, Kniele K, Corrigan JD. 2005. Patterns of alcohol use 1 year after traumatic brain injury: A population-based, epidemiological study. *Journal of the International Neuropsychological Society* 11(3):322-330.

Humana Military Healthcare Services. 2009. *About Humana military.* http://www.humana-military.com/AboutHMHS/about-us.asp. (Accessed July 28, 2009).

IOM (Institute of Medicine). 2007. *PTSD compensation and military service.* Washington, DC: The National Academies Press.

IOM. 2008. *Gulf War and health, Volume 6: Physiologic, psychologic and psychosocial effects of deployment-related stress.* Washington, DC: The National Academies Press.

Jacobson AM. 2001. Medically unexplained symptoms. In *Psychiatric secrets,* edited by Jacobson JL, Jacobson AM. Philadelphia: Hanley and Belfus.

Jaffee MS. 2009. Traumatic brain injury and the military health system. In *Systems engineering to improve traumatic brain injury care in the military health system: Workshop summary,* edited by Butler D, Buono J, Erdtmann F, and Reid P. Washington, DC: The National Academies Press.

Jensen PS, Martin D, Watanabe H. 1996. Children's response to parental separation during Operation Desert Storm. *Journal of the American Academy of Child & Adolescent Psychiatry* 35(4):433-441.

Jordan BK, Marmar CR, Fairbank JA, Schlenger WE, Kulka RA, Weiss DS. 1992. Problems in families of male Vietnam veterans with posttraumatic stress. *Journal of Consulting and Clinical Psychology* 60(6):916-926.

Judd LL, Akiskal HS, Maser JD, Zeller PJ, Endicott J, Coryell W, Paulus MP, Kunovac JL, Leon AC, Mueller TI, Rice JA, Keller MB. 1998. A prospective 12-year study of subsyndromal and syndromal depressive symptoms in unipolar major depressive disorders. *Archives of General Psychiatry* 55(8):694-700.

Kendler KS, Gallagher TJ, Abelson JM, Kessler RC. 1996. Lifetime prevalence, demographic risk factors, and diagnostic validity of nonaffective psychosis as assessed in a US community sample. The National Comorbidity Survey. *Archives of General Psychiatry* 53(11):1022-1031.

Kessler RC. 2004. The epidemiology of dual diagnosis. *Biological Psychiatry* 56(10): 730-737.

Kessler RC, Berglund P, Demler O, Jin R, Merikangas KR, Walters EE. 2005. Lifetime prevalence and age-of-onset distributions of DSM-IV disorders in the National Comorbidity Survey replication. *Archives of General Psychiatry* 62(6):593-603.

Killgore W, Melba DS, Stetz C, Castro CA, Hoge CW. 2006. The effects of prior combat experience on the expression of somatic and affective symptoms in deploying soldiers. *Journal of Psychosomatic Research* 60(4):379-385.

Kraus CA, Seignourel P, Balasubramanyam V, Snow AL, Wilson NL, Kunik ME, Schulz PE, Stanley MA. 2008. Cognitive-behavioral treatment for anxiety in patients with dementia: Two case studies. *Journal of Psychiatric Practice* 14(3):186-192.

Labutta R. 2009. Medical aspects of traumatic brain injury. In *Systems engineering to improve traumatic brain injury care in the military health system: Workshop summary,* edited by Butler D, Buono J, Erdtmann F, Reid P. Washington, DC: The National Academies Press.

Lapierre CB, Schwegler AF, Labauve BJ. 2007. Posttraumatic stress and depression symptoms in soldiers returning from combat operations in Iraq and Afghanistan. *Journal Trauma Stress* 20(6):933-943.

Lowenstein DH. 2009. Epilepsy after head injury: An overview. *Epilepsia* 50(s2):4-9.

Lurie N, Popkin M, Dysken M, Moscovice I, Finch M. 1992. Accuracy of diagnoses of schizophrenia in Medicaid claims. *Hospital and Community Psychiatry* 43(1):69-71.

Manguno-Mire G, Sautter F, Lyons J, Myers L, Perry D, Sherman M, Glynn S, Sullivan G. 2007. Psychological distress and burden among female partners of combat veterans with PTSD. *Journal of Nervous and Mental Disease* 195(2):144-151.

Marshall AD, Panuzio J, Taft CT. 2005. Intimate partner violence among military veterans and active duty service men. *Clinical Psychology Review* 25(7):862-876.

McCarroll JE, Ursano RJ, Fullerton CS, Liu X, Lundy A. 2002. Somatic symptoms in Gulf War mortuary workers. *Psychosomatic Medicine* 64(1):29-33.

Mehta KM, Ott A, Kalmijn S, Slooter AJ, van Duijn CM, Hofman A, Breteler MM. 1999. Head trauma and risk of dementia and Alzheimer's disease: The Rotterdam Study. *Neurology* 53(9):1959-1962.

MHAT (Mental Health Advisory Team-IV). 2006. *Operation Iraqi Freedom 05–07 final report.* November 17. Office of the Surgeon, Mutli-National Force Iraq and U.S. Army Surgeon General. http://www.armymedicine.army.mil/reports/mhat/mhat_iv/MHAT_IV_Report_17NOV06.pdf. (Accessed September 27, 2009).

Milliken CS, Auchterlonie JL, Hoge CW. 2009. Longitudinal assessment of mental health problems among active duty and reserve component soldiers returning from the Iraq War. *Journal of the American Medical Association* 298(18):2141-2148.

Moore DP, Jefferson JW. 2004a. Amnesia. In *Handbook of medical psychiatry*, 2nd ed. Philadelphia: Mosby.

Moore DP, Jefferson JW. 2004b. Delirium. In *Handbook of medical psychiatry*, 2nd ed. Philadelphia: Mosby.

Moore DP, Jefferson JW. 2004c. Dementia. In *Handbook of medical psychiatry*, 2nd ed. Philadelphia: Mosby.

Moore DP, Jefferson JW. 2004d. Personality change *Handbook of medical psychiatry*, 2nd ed. Philadelphia: Mosby.

Moore DP, Jefferson JW. 2004e. Schizophrenia. In *Handbook of medical psychiatry*, 2nd ed. Philadelphia: Mosby.

Moore DP, Jefferson JW. 2004f. Secondary depression. In *Handbook of medical psychiatry*, 2nd ed. Philadelphia: Mosby.

Nakase-Thompson R, Sherer M, Yablon SA, Nick TG, Trzepacz PT. 2004. Acute confusion following traumatic brain injury. *Brain Injury* 18(2):131-142.

National Military Family Association. 2006. *Statement of the National Military Family Association before the Department of Defense Task Force on Mental Health,* December 20. http://www.nmfa.org/site/DocServer/NMFA_DoD_Mental_health_Task_Force__12-20-06.pdf?docID=7701. (Accessed September 27, 2009).

Neighbors HW, Caldwell C, Williams DR, Nesse R, Taylor RJ, Bullard KM, Torres M, Jackson JS. 2007. Race, ethnicity, and the use of services for mental disorders: Results from the National Survey of American Life. *Archives of General Psychiatry* 64(4):485-494.

Newby JH, Ursano RJ, McCarroll JE, Martin LT, Norwood AE, Fullerton CS. 2003. Spousal aggression by U.S. Army female soldiers toward employed and unemployed civilian husbands. *American Journal of Orthopsychiatry* 73(3):288-293.

Niebuhr DW, Millikan AM, Cowan DN, Yolken R, Li Y, Weber NS. 2008. Selected infectious agents and risk of schizophrenia among U.S. military personnel. *American Journal of Psychiatry* 165(1):99-106.

NIMH (National Institute of Mental Health). 2009a. *Army study to assess risk and resilience in service members (Army STARRS).* http://www.nimh.nih.gov/health/topics/suicide-prevention/suicide-prevention-studies/army-study-to-assess-risk-and-resilience-in-service-members-army-starrs.shtml. (Accessed January 1, 2010).

NIMH. 2009b. *Depression.* http://www.nimh.nih.gov/health/publications/depression/complete-index.shtml. (Accessed June 22, 2009).

NRC (National Research Council). 2006. *Assessing fitness for military enlistment: Physical, medical, and mental health standards,* edited by Sackett PR, Mavor AS. Washington, DC: The National Academies Press.

Plassman BL, Havlik RJ, Steffens DC, Helms MJ, Newman TN, Drosdick D, Phillips C, Gau BA, Welsh-Bohmer KA, Burke JR, Guralnik JM, Breitner JC. 2000. Documented head injury in early adulthood and risk of Alzheimer's disease and other dementias. *Neurology* 55(8):1158-1166.

Reichman WE, Cummings JL. 2007. Dementia. In *Practice of geriatrics,* edited by Duthie EH Jr., Katz PR, Malone ML. Philadelphia: Saunders Elsevier.

Renshaw KD, Rodrigues CS, Jones DH. 2008. Psychological symptoms and marital satisfaction in spouses of Operation Iraqi Freedom veterans: Relationships with spouses' perceptions of veterans' experiences and symptoms. *Journal of Family Psychology* 22(4):586-594.

Rentz ED, Marshall SW, Loomis D, Casteel C, Martin SL, Gibbs D. 2007. Effect of deployment on the occurrence of child maltreatment in military and nonmilitary families. *American Journal of Epidemiology* 165(10):1199-1206.

Richardson RM. 2001. Dementia. In *Psychiatric secrets,* 2nd ed., edited by Jacobson JL, Jacobson AM. Philadelphia: Hanley and Belfus.

Rosenheck R, Fontana A. 1998. Warrior fathers and warrior sons: Intergenerational aspects of trauma. In *International handbook of multigenerational legacies of trauma,* edited by Danieli Y. New York: Plenum Press. Pp. 225-242.

Rosenheck R, Nathan P. 1985. Secondary traumatization in children of Vietnam veterans. *Hospital & Community Psychiatry* 36(5):538-539.

Rudolph JL, Marcantonio ER. 2007. Delirium. In *Practice of geriatrics,* edited by Duthie JEH, Katz PR, Malone ML. Philadelphia: Saunders Elsevier.

Sadler AG, Booth B, Nielson D, Doebbeling B. 2000. Health-related consequences of physical and sexual violence: Women in the military. *Obstetrics & Gynecology* 96(3):473-480.

Samper RE, Taft CT, King DW, King LA. 2004. Posttraumatic stress disorder symptoms and parenting satisfaction among a national sample of male Vietnam veterans. *Journal of Traumatic Stress* 11(4):311-315.

Sampson EL, Warren JD, Rossor MN. 2004. Young onset dementia. *Postgraduate Medical Journal* 80(941):125-139.

Sayer NA, Chiros CE, Sigford B, Scott S, Clothier B, Pickett T, Lew HL. 2008. Characteristics and rehabilitation outcomes among patients with blast and other injuries sustained during the global war on terror. *Archives of Physical Medicine and Rehabilitation* 89(1):163-170.

Seal KH, Metzler TJ, Gima, KS, Bertenthal D, Maguen S, Marmar CR. 2009. Trends and risk factors for mental health diagnoses among Iraq and Afghanistan veterans using Department of Veterans Affairs health care, 2002-2008. *American Journal of Public Health* 99(9):1651-1658.

Smith J, Seirafi J. 2006. Delirium and dementia. In *Rosen's emergency medicine: Concepts and clinical practice,* 6th ed., edited by Marx JA, Hockberger RS, Walls RM, Adams JG, Barsan WG, Biros MH, Danzl DF, Gausche-Hill M, Hamilton GC, Ling LJ, Newton EJ. Philadelphia: Mosby Elsevier.

Spencer SS. 2007. Seizures and epilepsy. In *Cecil medicine.* 23rd ed., edited by Goldman L, Ausiello D. Philadelphia: Saunders Elsevier.

Spettel CM, Wall TC, Allison J, Calhoun J, Kobylinski R, Fargason R, Kiefe CI. 2003. Identifying physician-recognized depression from administrative data: Consequences for quality measurement. *Health Services Research* 38(4):1081-1102.

St. Louis EK, Granner MA. 2008. Seizures and epilepsy in adolescents and adults. In *Conn's current therapy 2008,* 60th ed., edited by Rakel RE, Bope ET. Philadelphia: Saunders Elsevier.

Stover CS, Meadows AL, Kaufman J. 2009. Interventions for intimate partner violence: Review and implications for evidence-based practice. *Professional Psychology: Research and Practice* 40(3):223-233.

Street AE, Stafford J, Mahan CM, Hendricks A. 2008. Sexual harassment and assault experienced by reservists during military service: Prevalence and health correlates. *Journal of Rehabilitation Research & Development* 745(2):409-420.

Stuss DT, Binns MA, Carruth FG, Levine B, Brandys CE, Moulton RJ, Snow WG, Schwartz ML. 1999. The acute period of recovery from traumatic brain injury: Posttraumatic amnesia or posttraumatic confusional state? *Journal of Neurosurgery* 90(4):635-643.

Surís A, Lind L, Kashner M, Borman PD, Petty F. 2004. Sexual assault in women veterans: An examination of PTSD risk, health care utilization, and cost of care. *Psychosomatic Medicine* 66(5):749-756.

Tanielian T, Jaycox LH (Eds.). 2008. *Invisible wounds of war: Psychological and cognitive injuries, their consequences, and services to assist recovery.* Santa Monica, CA: RAND Corporation. http://www.rand.org/pubs/monographs/2008/RAND_MG720.pdf. (Accessed January 15, 2010).

TMA (TRICARE Management Activity). 2009. Data provided via e-mail from LCDR Richard Schobitz, OASD(HA)/TMA, in response to a request by the Committee on the Qualifications of Professionals Providing Mental Health Care Services Under TRICARE, July 27.

TriWest. 2009. *TriWest fast facts.* http://www.triwest.com/corporate/frames.aspx?page=/unauth/newContent/newAboutTriWest/default.asp. (Accessed July 28, 2009).

Unutzer J, Simon G, Pabiniak C, Bond K, Katon W. 1998. The treated prevalence of bipolar disorder in a large staff-model HMO. *Psychiatric Services* 49(8):1072-1078.

Unutzer J, Simon G, Pabiniak C, Bond K, Katon W. 2000. The use of administrative data to assess quality of care for bipolar disorder in a large staff model HMO. *General Hospital Psychiatry* 22(1):1-10.

VA/DOD (Department of Veterans Affairs/Department of Defense). 2004. *VA/DoD clinical practice guideline for management of post-traumatic stress, version 1.0.* Washington, DC: VA/DOD.

VA/DOD. 2009a. *VA/DoD clinical practice guideline for management of concussion/mild traumatic brain injury.* Washington, DC: VA/DOD.

VA/DOD. 2009b. *VA/DoD clinical practice guideline for management of major depressive disorder (MDD), version 2.0.* Washington, DC: VA/DOD.

VA/DOD. 2009c. *VA/DoD clinical practice guideline for management of substance use disorders (SUD), version 2.0.* Washington, DC: VA/DOD.

Vakil E. 2005. The effect of moderate to severe traumatic brain injury (TBI) on different aspects of memory: A selective review. *Journal of Clinical and Experimental Neuropsychology* 27(8):977-1021.

Wang PS, Lane M, Olfson M, Pincus HA, Wells KB, Kessler RC. 2005. Twelve-month use of mental health services in the United States: Results from the National Comorbidity Survey replication. *Archives of General Psychiatry* 62(6):629-640.

Wang PS, Demler O, Olfson M, Pincus HA, Wells KB, Kessler RC. 2006. Changing profiles of service sectors used for mental health care in the United States. *American Journal of Psychiatry* 163(7):1187-1198.

Warden D. 2006. Military TBI during the Iraq and Afghanistan wars. *Journal of Head Trauma Rehabilitation* 21(5):398-402.

Wortzel HS, Binswanger I, Anderson A, Adler L. 2009. Suicide among incarcerated veterans. *Journal of American Academy Psychiatry Law* 37(1):82-91.

Yehuda R, Flory JD, Southwick S, Charney D. 2006. Developing an agenda for translational studies of resilience and vulnerability following trauma exposure. *Annals of New York Academy of Science* 1071:379-396.

# 3

# Requirements Related to the Practice of Counseling

This chapter addresses several elements of the committee's task that pertain to how mental health counselors are trained and how they practice. It begins with a brief history of the profession of counseling and an overview of the education and training requirements for mental health professionals. It then provides details on how counselors are trained and on the accreditation of their educational institutions. Next, it introduces the primary means of professional recognition—licensing, credentialing, and privileging. Licensing requirements, including licensure examinations, are addressed, as are third-party certifications of professional standing. The chapter concludes with an examination of credentialing and privileging of counselors in TRICARE's direct-care and purchased-care systems and in the private sector. Box 3.1 at the end of the chapter contains a compilation of the abbreviations and acronyms used to denote the accrediting bodies, professional associations, certifications, and examinations referenced below.

Little has been published on the licensing, credentialing, and privileging of counselors; for that reason, the chapter provides detailed information on these topics.

## THE PROFESSION OF COUNSELING

A number of authors have published work on the history of the counseling profession (Bradley and Cox, 2001; Gibson and Mitchell,

2008; Hershenson and Berger, 2001; Remley and Herlihy, 2010; Sweeney, 2001). That information is summarized here.

In the 1950s, the psychology profession was establishing the doctoral level as the requirement for professional status, and counseling psychology was developing as a specialty within psychology. Historical events were leading to the rapid development of school counseling programs and vocational-rehabilitation counseling. Eventually, changes in counseling psychology, the school-counseling movement, and federal funding of vocational-rehabilitation counseling led to the emergence of the new profession of counseling.

At the beginning of its effort to become a profession, psychology recognized people who had master's degrees as professional psychologists. The American Psychological Association (APA) declared in the 1950s that in the future only psychologists who held doctoral degrees would be recognized as professionals. The profession decided to continue to recognize all current psychologists who held master's degrees and allow them to practice but in the future to allow into the profession only those who held doctoral degrees in psychology. Licensure laws in psychology throughout the United States were changed to reflect the new position.

In 1957, when the Soviet Union successfully orbited the first spacecraft, Sputnik, politicians in the United States feared that, inasmuch as the Soviet Union had exceeded American technology and beaten the United States in the "race to space," it might overpower the United States politically as well. In response to that fear, Congress created substantial programs to encourage young people to seek careers in technical and scientific fields. The effort included placing counselors in high schools to channel students into mathematics and science courses. Throughout the United States, universities created summer institutes in which high-school teachers were given basic courses that led to their placement in high schools as guidance counselors. In most instances, high-school teachers were given two or three courses in guidance or counseling, which allowed them to be certified as school counselors and to assume guidance-counselor positions in schools. Because the primary purpose of the effort was to encourage students to take mathematics and science courses, it did not seem necessary for counselors to be prepared beyond the training provided in the summer institutes.

School-accreditation groups were soon requiring high schools to have guidance counselors if they were to receive or continue their accreditation. Today, middle-school and high-school accreditation requires that schools have counselors, and in some areas elementary schools are required to have them. For school counselors to be certified, almost all states now require them to have received master's degrees and to have completed specified courses and an internship.

An emphasis on rehabilitation of wounded soldiers began as early as the Revolutionary War. However, the modern era of rehabilitation began between 1900 and 1930 with increasing concern about the well-being of industrially disabled persons and the establishment of state and federal rehabilitation services. After increased concern about veterans of World War II and other people who had disabilities by the 1950s, there was recognition in the United States that citizens who had physical or mental disabilities were not being given the help that they needed to become productive members of society in that they were not receiving services by specifically trained rehabilitation counselors. As a result, legislation was passed in 1954 that established master's-level rehabilitation counseling programs and provided counseling and educational resources that were meant to help persons who had disabilities to function more autonomously (Sales, 2007).

A major component of the legislation was funding to prepare counselors to help people to evaluate their disabilities, to make plans to work, and to find satisfactory employment. As a result of the funding, new master's degree programs in rehabilitation counseling were developed, and existing programs were expanded. State rehabilitation agencies created positions in rehabilitation case management and counseling for the graduates of the programs.

The dynamics of the creation of the specialty of counseling psychology, the decision in the psychology profession to recognize professionals only at the doctoral level, the emergence of school counseling, and the funding of vocational-rehabilitation counseling programs led to the creation of counseling as a separate master's degree–level profession. The origins of the profession were in the convergence of several disparate forces rather than in a single event.

Changes that have taken place in the last 20–30 years in the field of counseling include the lengthening of most educational programs from 30 to 48 to 60 semester hours in some specialties, professionalization of counseling through credentialing and legislation, the passage of laws granting privileged communication to interactions between counselors and their clients, and increases in the body of knowledge specific to counseling, as distinguished from other mental health professions, through scholarly writing.

Counseling has made progress toward recognition as a profession at a rate comparable with that of professionalization efforts in other mental health disciplines, such as psychology. Connecticut became the first state to pass a law licensing psychologists in 1945, and licensing laws for psychologists had been enacted in all 50 states when Missouri passed its law in 1977, 32 years later (Benjamin, 2006). In comparison, the first counselor-licensure bill was passed in Virginia in 1976, and all 50 states had passed licensure bills for counselors by 2009, 33 years later.

## Distinctions Between Counselors and Other Mental Health Professionals

Table 3.1 summarizes the similarities and differences in educational and training requirements among the mental health professions recognized by TRICARE. It was adapted from a summary by Remley and Herlihy (2010) that was based on information provided by the organizations that accredit the listed professions: for counseling, the Council for Accreditation of Counseling and Related Educational Programs (CACREP, 2008); for pastoral counselors, the American Association of Pastoral Counselors (AAPC, 2009); for marriage and family therapy, the American Association for Marriage and Family Therapy (AAMFT, 2004); for social work, the Council on Social Work Education (CSWE, 2008); for nursing, the Commission on Collegiate Nursing Education (CCNE, 2009); for psychology, the APA Commission on Accreditation (APA CoA, 2008); and for psychiatry, the Liaison Committee on Medical Education (LCME, 2008) and the Accreditation Council for Graduate Medical Education (ACGME, 2007).

The 2006 IOM report *Improving the Quality of Health Care for Mental and Substance-Use Conditions: Quality Chasm Series* addresses the education of mental health professionals in far greater detail, and offers recommendations for increasing workforce capacity.

## How Counselors Are Trained and Practice

The evolution of counseling began with the development of counseling specialties that were formed to meet the needs of particular employment settings, types of client populations, or even techniques

**TABLE 3.1** Comparison of Preparation Requirements for the Mental Health Professions

| Profession and Graduate Education Required | Summary of Required Courses and Required Supervised Field Experience |
|---|---|
| **Counseling**<br>48–60 graduate credits required for master's degree | Graduate coursework required in professional identity; social, cultural diversity; human growth, development; career development; helping relationships; group work; assessment; research, program evaluation; specialty (mental health counseling, community counseling, school counseling, career counseling, marriage and family counseling and therapy, college counseling, gerontologic counseling, student affairs)<br><br>100-hour practicum, 600-hour internship required |
| **Pastoral Counseling** | Field of pastoral counseling does not accredit academic preparation programs; people may become certified as pastoral counselors by American Association of Pastoral Counselors, but academic preparation programs not accredited |
| **Marriage and Family Therapy**<br>Minimum number of graduate credits not specified | Graduate coursework required that covers 128 competencies in six domains: admission to treatment; clinical assessment, diagnosis; treatment planning, case management; therapeutic interventions; legal issues, ethics, standards; research, program evaluation<br><br>Number of hours of practicum, internship not specified |
| **Social Work**<br>60 graduate credits required for master's degree | Coursework required in professional social worker identity; ethical principles; critical thinking; diversity, difference; advancing human rights, social and economic justice; research-informed practice, practice-informed research; human behavior, social environment; policy practice; contexts that shape practice; engaging, assessing, intervening, evaluating individuals, families, groups, organizations, communities<br><br>Minimum of 900 hours of field experience required |

*continued*

**TABLE 3.1** Continued

| Profession and Graduate Education Required | Summary of Required Courses and Required Supervised Field Experience |
|---|---|
| **Nursing**<br>Minimum number of graduate credits not specified | Graduate nursing coursework in research; policy, organization, financing of health care; ethics; professional role development; theoretical foundations of nursing practice; human diversity, social issues; health promotion, disease prevention; advanced health, physical assessment; advanced physiology, pathophysiology; advanced pharmacology; psychiatric nursing<br><br>Minimum of 500 hours of direct clinical practice<br><br>(Additional requirements are placed on persons practicing in psychiatric nurse specialties) |
| **Psychology**<br>3 full-time years of graduate study required for doctoral degree | Graduate coursework required in biological aspects of behavior; cognitive, affective aspects of behavior; social aspects of behavior; history, systems of psychology; psychological measurement; research methodology; techniques of data analysis; individual differences in behavior; human development; dysfunctional behavior or psychopathology; professional standards, ethics; theories, methods of assessment, diagnosis; effective intervention; consultation, supervision; evaluating efficacy of interventions; cultural, individual diversity; attitudes essential for life-long learning, scholarly inquiry, professional problem solving<br><br>1 full-time year of residency required |

**TABLE 3.1** Continued

| Profession and Graduate Education Required | Summary of Required Courses and Required Supervised Field Experience |
|---|---|
| **Psychiatry**<br>130 weeks required for medical degree (usually 4 years) | MD requires coursework in anatomy; biochemistry; genetics; physiology; microbiology, immunology; pathology; pharmacology, therapeutics; preventive medicine; scientific method; accurate observation of biomedical phenomena; critical analysis of data; organ systems; preventive, acute, chronic, continuing, rehabilitative, end-of-life care; clinical experiences in primary care, family medicine, internal medicine, obstetrics and gynecology, pediatrics, psychiatry, surgery in outpatient, inpatient settings; multidisciplinary content, such as emergency medicine, geriatrics; disciplines that support general medical practice, such as diagnostic imaging, clinical pathology; clinical, translational research, including how such research is conducted, evaluated, explained to patients, applied to patient care; communication skills as related to physician responsibilities, including communication with patients, families, colleagues, other health professionals; addressing medical consequences of common societal problems, for example, providing instruction in diagnosis, prevention, appropriate reporting, treatment of people for violence, abuse; how people of diverse cultures, belief systems perceive health, illness and respond to various symptoms, diseases, treatments; sex, cultural biases; medical ethics, human values<br><br>Psychiatry residency curriculum must include patient care; medical knowledge; practice-based patient learning, improvement; interpersonal, communication skills; professionalism; systems-based practice; research; required topics include supervised practice in providing psychiatric services to diverse populations<br><br>48-month residency in psychiatry is required, which includes 12-month internship in primary-care clinical setting |

SOURCE: Adapted from Remley and Herlihy (2010).

rather than with the establishment of a general strong central profession with a logical metastructure before specialties were elaborated (Hosie, 1995; Myers, 1995; Sweeney, 1995). That historical pattern heavily influenced the structure of counselor education, training, and practice (Myers, 1995). As a result, there is a need to understand and differentiate between the various types of specialty education and practice so that they may be clearly related to the specific practice of mental health counseling at the independently licensed level. Academic degrees in counseling indicate a graduate's specialty and need to be related to the graduate's field of practice (Schweiger et al., 2008).

### *Training and Education*

**Overview** People enter the profession of counseling through obtaining a master's or doctoral degree in counseling from a counselor educational program or a related program (such as a rehabilitation counseling program). There are no standard requirements for a specific type of undergraduate degree, and undergraduate preparation requirements depend on the educational institution. Master's degree preparation includes a practicum and internship in the specialty. Two bodies recognized by the American Counseling Association (ACA) accredit counselor educational programs: CACREP, which provides accreditation in a variety of counseling specialties other than rehabilitation counseling, and the Council on Rehabilitation Education (CORE), which accredits only rehabilitation counselor educational programs. Both bodies are recognized by the Council for Higher Education Accreditation (CHEA).

Because the two groups are substantially similar in their goals, objectives, and core knowledge and competence, they engaged in serious discussions about a possible merger in the mid-2000s but decided not to continue active pursuit of a merger at the time. The two organizations accredit most of the counselor educational programs, but some related specialties, such as pastoral counseling, are not accredited by them.

Not all counselor educational programs are accredited, but the proportion of such programs that are accredited continues to increase. Programs that are not accredited generally have patterned their curriculum requirements after the CACREP core curriculum requirements because many states that license counselors require curricula that are based on the CACREP standards even if they do not specifically require CACREP accreditation (ACA, 2008).

As noted previously, the profession of counseling evolved in its early years through interdisciplinary influences and in response to the needs of clients in various employment settings. The overall definition of the profession has thus developed emphases both on personal growth and a wellness perspective and on providing counseling to people who have mental disorders. Those emphases permit practitioners in counseling to understand and work with problems as diverse as vocational decision-making for people in the ordinary course of their lives and interpretation and diagnosis of substantial symptoms and treatment options for people who have mental disorders (Gladding, 2009). The different emphases can be said to be reflected in the differences between the 2001 CACREP standards in community counseling that emphasized preventive development and the mental health counseling specialty accreditation that emphasized diagnosis of and treatment for mental health disorders (Chronister et al., 2009). Those two specialties have long been seen as closely related since their inception and were originally thought to assist in differentiating preparation needed by counselors who would work in community-based agencies (Community Counseling) from that needed by those who would work in private-practice settings (Mental Health Counseling).

The profession has moved toward a more consolidated view of how elements of the specialties are related to one another, and the 2009 CACREP accreditation standards consolidated the two specialties most closely related to the practice of mental health counseling—Community Counseling and Mental Health Counseling—into the singular category of Clinical Mental Health Counseling (CACREP, 2009a). In practice, it has been possible for graduates of the programs to apply for licensure and work in either type of setting because of the similarity of the types of work. That was the case even though counselors educated in Community Counseling programs typically took the mental health courses either as pregraduation electives or after graduation and then fulfilled the additional types and hours of supervised practice required (Neukrug, 2003).

Since the consolidated standards for Clinical Mental Health Counseling went into effect on July 1, 2009, all programs that were accredited in Community Counseling or Mental Health Counseling before then have had to renew their accreditation in the new category when reaccreditation became necessary. That change standardized accreditation requirements in many ways, including moving all programs in the category to a minimum of 60 semester hours and requiring clinical coursework for most accredited counseling programs. The Clinical Mental Health Counseling curriculum has a heavy emphasis on clinical counseling and requires demonstration of skills and practices in the foundations of counseling, counseling, prevention and intervention, diversity and advocacy, assessment, research and evaluation, and diagnosis (CACREP, 2009a).

**Number and types of programs** As of August 2009, CACREP accredited 569 master's and doctoral level counseling programs in 239 institutions in the following fields: 164 in Community Counseling; 55 in Counselor Education and Supervision; 19 in College Counseling; 9 in Career Counseling; 2 in Gerontologic Counseling; 32 in Marital, Couple, and Family Counseling and Therapy; 63 in Mental Health Counseling; 22 in Student Affairs; 2 in Student Affairs Practice in Higher Education with emphasis on College Counseling; and 201 in School Counseling (CACREP, 2009c). About 100 other master's programs for rehabilitation counselors are accredited by CORE (2009c).

In an April 2009 presentation to the committee, CACREP Executive Director Carol Bobby (2009) noted that CACREP's expectation is that most existing Community and Mental Health Counseling programs will make the transition to the new single standard on the basis of two recent surveys that the organization undertook to assess preparedness to meet the 60-semester-hours requirement. If that expectation is realized, there will be over 200 accredited Clinical Mental Health Counseling Programs (Bobby, 2009); this number would exceed the number of school counseling.

A number of non–CACREP-accredited programs also offer Community Counseling and Mental Health Counseling degrees. In 2001, Altekruse et al. reported that 84 out of 205 Community Counseling and 58 out of 79 Mental Health Counseling programs were not CACREP accredited; it is not known how many of the programs remain unaccredited by that organization.

**Admission and graduation requirements** Schools vary in the requirements placed on entrants into their graduate educational programs in counseling. Admission requirements include a bachelor's degree and some combination of minimum grade-point average and standardized test scores, successful completion of relevant preparatory coursework (typically in psychology), letters of recommendation, personal interviews, and evidence of interest in the field as evinced by volunteer work and the like (Schweiger et al., 2008). ACA notes that "majors in education, sociology, psychology, or any of the social sciences can be very helpful in graduate study," but no specific undergraduate degree is required (ACA, 2009). Institutions set their own policies regarding whether, or the conditions under which, they recognize undergraduate coursework for completion of graduate-degree requirements.

Entry-level master's programs are typically 2 years long. Graduation requirements typically mirror the requirements to apply for licensure as a mental health counselor in the state where the school is. They include successful completion of core curricula and a minimum course, practicum, and related training and experience hours. Depending on the institution, students may also need to pass comprehensive written or oral examinations, complete a thesis, or turn in a portfolio (Schweiger et al., 2008).

Similar statements could be made about master's-level professional programs in the other mental health disciplines.

**Location of programs** As a result of the historically strong connections between guidance counseling and education in traditions and institutions, most counselor educational programs are in colleges and schools of education (Sweeney, 2001).

**Curricular content** The two credentialing bodies in counseling (CACREP and CORE) and the two major certification bodies for counselors (the National Board for Certified Counselors [NBCC] and the Commission on Rehabilitation Counselor Certification [CRCC]) have identified the same eight categories of core knowledge for professional counselors: professional identity, social and cultural diversity, human growth and development, career development, helping relationships, group work, assessment, and research and program evaluation (Chronister et al., 2009). These categories are supplemented in each specialty with additional categories of knowledge as established by the program accreditation body. In its 2009 standards, CACREP added demonstration of skills and practices specifically in each of the knowledge categories, thus requiring a competence-based approach to evaluating programs (CACREP, 2009a). CACREP and CORE also impose the same clinical training and internship requirements; these are specified below.

### *Practice*

**Overview** According to the US Department of Labor (DOL) *Occupational Outlook Handbook*, counselors held about 638,100 jobs in the United States in 2008. They worked in the following specialties: 275,800 educational, vocational, and school counseling; 129,500 rehabilitation counseling; 113,300 mental health counseling; 86,100 substance-abuse and behavioral-disorder counseling; and 33,400 counseling in other fields (BLS, 2009-10).

Bureau of Labor Statistics projections show the employment market for counselors growing at an above-average rate of 18% from 2008 to 2018. Although the specialties of counseling are projected to grow at various rates, the employment growth rate for mental health counselors is projected to be 24%. DOL attributes the latter rate to increases in the staffing, the increasing approval of counselors for reimbursement by insurance and managed-care companies, and increased demand as persons become more willing to seek help for mental health issues (BLS, 2009-10).

**Job settings after graduation** All graduates of counselor education have the core identity of and education in counseling, but most counselors find employment that is consistent with the specialization in which they were trained. Schweiger et al. (2008) found that master's-level graduates of counselor educational programs found employment as follows: 67% of community-counseling and 65% of the mental health–counseling graduates in agencies, 94% of school-counseling graduates in schools, and 69% of college-counseling graduates in higher-education and student-affairs settings. Private practice as an employment setting occurs at lower rates: 10% of college counselors, 11% of community counselors, 8% of school counselors, and 12% of mental health counselors (Schweiger et al., 2008).

In 2004, the US Department of Health and Human Services reported the main primary work settings of 100,533 professional mental health counselors on whom information was available: academic setting,

33.4% (universities, colleges, and elementary and secondary schools); clinic, 22.5% (mental health and other health clinics); other and not specified, 16.0%; and individual practice, 15.1%. Those four categories account for 87% of the work environments reported by the clinically trained counselors (Manderscheid and Berry, 2004).

## ACCREDITATION OF COUNSELOR EDUCATIONAL INSTITUTIONS

Voluntary accreditation in higher education is a collegial process of self-assessment and peer review for improvement of academic quality and public accountability of institutions and programs. CHEA characterizes accreditation as "the primary means of assuring and improving the quality of higher education institutions and programs in the United States" (CHEA, 2009). This quality-review process occurs on a periodic basis, usually every 3–10 years. Typically, it involves three major activities:

1. Self-study by an institution or program using the standards or criteria of an accrediting organization.
2. Peer review of an institution or program to gather evidence and validate what has been provided in documents, observation of activities, and inspection of records that could not be accomplished in the document review.
3. Decision or judgment by an accrediting organization to accredit, accredit with conditions, or not accredit an institution or program.

Generally speaking, there are two types of higher-education accreditation: institutional and specialized. Institutional accreditation is granted by regional and national accrediting commissions; these accrediting bodies are recognized by the US Department of Education (ED)—for institutions that have a "federal purpose"—or through a voluntary recognition process administered by CHEA. Specialized accreditation is awarded to professional academic programs in institutions or to occupational schools that offer specific training and knowledge; these accrediting bodies are also recognized by ED or CHEA.

## Council for Accreditation of Counseling and Related Educational Programs

CACREP is an independent accrediting agency created by ACA. It was incorporated in 1981. Institutional, curricular, and other requirements for CACREP accreditation of educational programs are described below.

For a program to be eligible for CACREP accreditation review, the institution that houses the program must be accredited by one of the regional or national institutional accrediting bodies recognized by CHEA. The institution and the program must also have appropriate institutional and faculty support; the academic unit overseeing the program must have at least three core faculty members whose academic appointments are in counselor education.

The CACREP accreditation cycle is for 8 years unless there are some minor deficiencies. A 2-year accreditation is granted to programs that substantially meet the requirements for accredited status but that need to address relatively minor standards-related deficiencies (CACREP, 2009b).

Academic-hours requirements vary by specialty. Those for Clinical Mental Health Counseling were established in 2009 and reflect a transition period for programs that were previously accredited in Community Counseling, which required 48 graduate semester hours. As of July 1, 2009, 54 graduate semester credit hours or 81 quarter credit hours were required. As of July 1, 2013, 60 graduate semester credit hours or 90 quarter credit hours—the standard already in place for accredited Mental Health Counseling programs—will be required (CACREP, 2009a).

Students must complete 100 clock hours over a minimum 10-week academic term. The 100 clock hours must include 40 clock hours of direct service with actual clients that contribute to the development of counseling skills. Specific individual and group supervision is required. One hour a week is required for individual or triadic supervision by a program faculty member. An average of 1½ hours per week is required for group supervision by a program faculty member or a student supervisor.

The supervised internship program requires completion of 600 clock hours in the student's designated program field. The internship is begun after successful completion of a practicum. At least 240 clock hours of direct service, which must include leading groups, is required. Individual and triadic supervision is usually performed by the onsite clinical supervisor. Group supervision is performed by a program faculty member.

CACREP also specifies standards for persons serving as individual or group practicum or internship supervisors.

According to the 12th edition of *Counselor Preparation*, a reference text on educational programs, "the goal of most [internship] programs is to provide an in-depth experience at a site that has working conditions similar to the student's career goals." However, there is no requirement for students to have experiences in specific mental health diagnostic categories (Schweiger et al., 2008).

### *Clinical Mental Health Counseling*

Clinical Mental Health Counseling curricula have the following sections: foundations; counseling, prevention, and intervention; diversity and advocacy; assessment; research and evaluation; and diagnosis. Each section is supported by learning outcomes related to knowledge, skills, and practices. There is also a set of "common core curricular experiences and demonstrated knowledge" requirements shared by all the counseling specialties that CACREP accredits. The following is a sample of relevant skills and practices associated with Clinical Mental Health Counseling (CACREP, 2009b):

*Counseling, Prevention, and Intervention*

- Uses the principles and practices of diagnosis, treatment, referral, and prevention of mental and emotional disorders to initiate, maintain, and terminate counseling.
- Demonstrates the ability to use procedures for assessing and managing suicide risk.
- Knows the disease concept and etiology of addiction and co-occurring disorders.
- Provides appropriate counseling strategies when working with clients with addiction and co-occurring disorders.
- Demonstrates the ability to recognize his or her own limitations as a clinical mental health counselor and to seek supervision or refer clients when appropriate.

*Diversity and Advocacy*

- Understands how living in a multicultural society affects clients who are seeking clinical mental health counseling services.

- Demonstrates the ability to modify counseling systems, theories, techniques, and interventions to make them culturally appropriate for diverse populations.

*Assessment*

- Selects appropriate comprehensive assessment interventions to assist in diagnosis and treatment planning, with an awareness of cultural bias in the implementation and interpretation of assessment protocols.
- Demonstrates skill in conducting an intake interview, a mental status evaluation, a biopsychosocial history, a mental health history, and a psychological assessment for treatment planning and caseload management.
- Screens for addiction, aggression, and danger to self and/or others, as well as co-occurring mental disorders.
- Understands basic classifications, indications, and contraindications of commonly prescribed psychopharmacological medications so that appropriate referrals can be made for medication evaluations and so that the side effects of such medications can be identified.
- Applies the assessment of a client's stage of dependence, change, or recovery to determine the appropriate treatment modality and placement criteria within the continuum of care.

*Diagnosis*

- Demonstrates appropriate use of diagnostic tools, including the current edition of the *DSM* (*Diagnostic and Statistical Manual of Mental Disorders*) to describe the symptoms and clinical presentation of clients with mental and emotional impairments.
- Is able to conceptualize an accurate multiaxial diagnosis of disorders presented by a client and discuss the differential diagnosis with collaborating professionals.
- Differentiates between diagnosis and developmentally appropriate reactions during crises, disasters, and other trauma-causing events.

The language used to express the learning outcomes calls into question whether the skills and practices would support some of the knowledge and skills to practice independently in circumstances that would include diagnosis of complex clinical conditions. The lack of specificity of the learning outcomes and the use of such words as "assist," "screen," and "collaborate" give the impression that the preparation may not by itself be adequate to support independent practice. It should be noted, however, that these are learning outcomes on graduation from an accredited CACREP academic program and before the generally required 2-year clinical experience that precedes licensing. That is consistent with patterns noted among the mental health professions. The Annapolis Coalition on the Behavioral Health Workforce has observed that graduate education and training for all mental health professionals lack specificity in a number of knowledge and competence elements that are essential for professional contemporary mental health practice (Hoge et al., 2002). The presence of the terms "assist" and "collaborating" can also been seen as being consistent with the calls for preparation to engage in collaborative approaches to practice (Hoge et al., 2002).

## Council on Rehabilitation Education

The mission of CORE is the accreditation of rehabilitation-counselor education (RCE) programs to promote the effective delivery of rehabilitation services to people who have disabilities by promoting and fostering continuing review and improvement of master's degree–level RCE programs. It is an independent accrediting agency that was incorporated in 1972 by a group of rehabilitation professionals.

CORE accredits graduate master's degree programs that provide academic preparation for professional RCE. It also maintains a registry of programs that meet curriculum and outcome standards or guidelines for undergraduate programs in rehabilitation.

CORE has two commissions: the Commission on Standards and Accreditation and the Commission on Undergraduate Education. The Commission on Standards and Accreditation is the evaluation component of CORE. It has the responsibility of evaluating programs for compliance with CORE standards and recommending the type of accreditation recognition. There are two types of recognition. Candidacy for accreditation is granted to academic programs that are in the early stages but comply with all the standards except performance of graduates. Full accreditation provides evidence that a program complies with all standards and is able to maintain that level of compliance through the duration of the recognition. The latter recognition includes objective assessment of the professional performance of graduates. As of October 2009, there were 97 fully accredited programs and 11 programs that were candidates for accreditation (CORE, 2010).

The Commission on Undergraduate Education is responsible for recommendation to CORE of standards and criteria required for the undergraduate registry.

The eligibility criteria for any academic program to be considered for either type of recognition are as follows:

- The educational institution is accredited by the appropriate regional accreditation body and offers graduate degrees in fields other than that being evaluated.
- The program provides for 2 years of full-time graduate study.
- The program has institutional approval for courses and degrees offered.
- The program has a person designated as coordinator, or the equivalent, who is a Certified Rehabilitation Counselor.
- The program has a written statement of its mission, objectives, curriculum, and criteria for student selection.

### *General Curriculum Requirements, Knowledge Domains, and Educational Outcomes*

There are 10 knowledge domains with related outcomes:

1. Professional identity.
2. Social and cultural diversity.
3. Human growth and development.
4. Employment and career development.
5. Counseling and consultation.
6. Group work.
7. Assessment.
8. Research and program evaluation.
9. Medical, functional, and environmental aspects of disability.
10. Rehabilitation service and resources.

Specific selected outcomes in several knowledge domains are related to practice in mental health (CORE, 2008a):

*Counseling and Consultation*

- Conduct individual counseling sessions with consumers.
- Establish in collaboration with the consumer, individual counseling goals and objectives.
- Assist the consumer with crisis resolution.
- Recommend strategies to assist the consumer in solving identified problems that may impede the rehabilitation process.
- Explain the implications of assessment/evaluation results on planning and decision making.
- Assist the consumer in developing acceptable work behavior.
- Adjust counseling approaches or styles to meet the needs of individual consumers.
- Terminate counseling relationships with consumers in a manner that enhances their ability to function independently.
- Recognize consumers who demonstrate psychological problems (e.g., depression, suicidal ideation) and refer when appropriate.
- Interpret diagnostic information (e.g., vocational and educational tests, records, and medical data) to the consumer.
- Assist consumers to successfully deal with situations involving conflict resolution and behavior management.

*Group Work*

- Articulate the principles of group dynamics with persons with disabilities including group process components, developmental state theories, group members' roles and behaviors, and therapeutic factors of group work.
- Facilitate the group process with the individual's family/significant others, including advocates.
- Apply approaches used for other types of group work with persons with disabilities including skill groups, psychoeducational groups, and group counseling.
- Apply theories of group counseling when working with persons with disabilities including commonalities, distinguishing characteristics, and pertinent research and literature.

- Apply group counseling methods including group counselor orientation and behaviors, appropriate referral and selection criteria, and methods of evaluation and effectiveness.

*Assessment*

- Determine an individual's eligibility for rehabilitation services and/or programs.
- Utilize assessment information to determine appropriate services.
- Assess the unique strengths, resources, and experiences of an individual, including career knowledge and interests.
- Assess an individual's vocational or independent living skills, aptitudes, interests, and preferences.
- Use behavioral observations to make inferences about work personality, characteristics, and adjustment.

*Medical, Functional, and Environmental Aspects of Disability*

- Explain basic medical aspects of the human body system and disabilities.
- Explain functional capacity implications of medical and psychosocial information.
- Apply working knowledge of the impact of disability on the individual, the family, and the environment.
- Consult with medical professionals regarding functional capacities, prognosis, and treatment for consumers.

### *Educational and Clinical-Experience Requirements*

The 2008 CORE program standards require a minimum of 48 semester hours for RCE programs, but if the state in which the program exists requires 60 semester hours for licensure, the program must identify and provide the additional 12 semester hours required for licensure (CORE, 2008b).

Students are required to have a minimum of 100 hours of supervised rehabilitation counseling practicum with at least 40 hours of direct service to persons who have disabilities. The supervised rehabilitation-counseling internship involves 600 hours of applied experience in an agency or programs, including at least 240 hours of direct service to people who have disabilities. Both the practicum and the internship require 1 hour per week of individual supervision or 1½ hours per week of group (no more than 10 students/group) supervision by a program faculty member or another qualified person who works in cooperation with a program faculty member. There is no requirement for students to have experience with specific mental health diagnostic categories.

The academic preparation for a Rehabilitation Counselor does not, in the committee's view, support diagnostic and treatment ability in mental health associated with specific psychopathologic conditions unless additional coursework and clinical experiences are obtained, as would be the case when rehabilitation counselors become licensed as mental health counselors in states that require such additional courses and postgraduate clinical practice.

### The Concept of "CACREP Equivalence"

"CACREP-equivalent" is a designation used by educational institutions and agencies, such as state licensure boards,[1] to denote an academic or training program that ostensibly meets the student-outcome accreditation requirements of CACREP but that does not have formal recognition from CACREP.

The concept of CACREP equivalence appears to be based on substantially equivalent numbers of semester hours or quarter hours in an accredited institution. An unknown proportion of applicants who present coursework to be evaluated for CACREP equivalence are rehabilitation counselors who have graduated from one of the roughly 100 CORE-accredited programs.

Most licensure bodies that provide for equivalent coursework require specific course content in designated program areas that are consistent with the CACREP core curriculum. There appears to be little attempt to evaluate learning outcomes, and there is no specific documented evidence to indicate how equivalence is determined. In addition, because of the wide variation among courses, course titles,

---

[1]For example, the Code of Alabama § 34-8A-7(4) ("Qualifications of applicants for professional counselor license") states "the applicant has received a master's degree from a regionally accredited institution of higher learning which is primarily professional counseling in content based on national standards *or the substantial equivalent in both subject matter and extent of training*. The board shall use the standards of nationally recognized professional counseling associations as guides in establishing the standards for counselor licensure" (emphasis added).

and qualifications of instructors, there is no empirical evidence that other accepted courses of study by licensure bodies have the same learning outcomes as accredited CACREP Clinical Mental Health Counseling programs.

## MEANS OF PROFESSIONAL RECOGNITION

Recognition as a qualified mental health practitioner and the ability to provide mental health services in the US health-care system typically has three tiers. The first tier is licensure in one's discipline in the state in which one practices, the second is credentialing, and the third is the granting of appropriate clinical privileges to diagnose mental health disorders or treat those who are experiencing them. Credentialing and privileging are considered critical elements in ensuring the delivery of high-quality mental health care because they involve verification of completed licensure requirements and assessment of a provider's competence to deliver high-quality care to beneficiaries.

Licensure is granted by a state; it takes the form of a license, certification, or registration and refers to official or legal permission to practice in the state. Credentialing is the systematic process of screening and evaluating qualifications and other forms of professional recognition, such as licensure, education, training, and clinical experience to ensure that specific requirements are met. Overall, the credentialing process aims to ensure that a person is able to perform according to specified standards (Department of Veterans Affairs, 2008). Privileging is the process by which the scope and content of patient-care services are defined for an individual provider. Privileging by a health-care organization is based on an evaluation of a person's credentials and performance in delivering services, and it authorizes a person to perform the duties outlined in his or her professional scope of practice.

Clinical privileging is the process by which a licensed independent practitioner is granted permission by law and a health-care facility to practice independently and to provide specific services within the scope of practice defined by the practitioner's license. It is based on individual competence to provide services and is both facility-specific and provider-specific (HHS, 1996). Department of Defense Directive 6025.13 states that clinical privileges are to be "based on the capability of the healthcare facility, licensure, relevant training and experience, current competence, health status, judgment, and peer and department head recommendations" (DOD, 1995).

The Military Health System also uses the term *current competence* in reference to the capabilities of health-care providers. It defines the term as follows (DOD, 2004):

> DL1.1.10. Current Competence. The state of having adequate ability to perform the functions of a practitioner in a particular discipline as measured by meeting the following:
>
> DL1.1.10.1. Authorized to practice a specified scope of care under a written plan of supervision at any time within the past 2 years; or, completed formal graduate professional education in a specified clinical specialty at any time within the past 2 years; or, privileged to practice a specified scope of care at any time within the past 2 years.
>
> DL1.1.10.2. Actively pursued the practice of his or her discipline within the past 2 years by having encountered a sufficient number of clinical cases to represent a broad spectrum of the privileges requested; and,
>
> DL1.1.10.3. Satisfactorily practiced the discipline as determined by the results of professional staff monitoring and evaluation of the quality and appropriateness of patient care.

## LICENSING

### Overview

All states, the District of Columbia, Puerto Rico, and Guam license mental health counselors. Several states used a tiered licensure system that includes an associate-counselor level and a general-counselor level. Other states differentiate between standard professional counselors and clinical professional counselors; scopes of practice are delineated according to the licensure level.

Typically, in states that have multiple levels of licensure, independent diagnosis and treatment can be performed only by those at the higher level. For example, licensure in Arkansas includes a level for associate counselors and a level for professional counselors. Only licensed professional counselors are allowed to diagnose and to treat patients. In Kansas, licensed professional counselors may practice only under the supervision of a licensed clinical professional counselor. Illinois's licensure of clinical professional counselors authorizes the independent private practice of clinical professional counseling whereas licensure of professional counselors authorizes only the general practice of professional counseling.

Further information on the various licenses granted by states and on the scope of practice associated with each license can be found in Appendix G. In response to elements of the statement of task, the table that makes up that appendix includes data on license names and associated educational, clinical-experience, and other licensing requirements; on licensure renewal and continuing education requirements; on independent-practice strictures; and on coverage of care by health insurance.

## License Requirements

### *Education*

Most states require master's level–licensed counselors to complete a minimum of 48 semester hours of coursework in an accredited program in addition to various numbers of hours in a practicum and internship. There is no single accepted standard, but most states use or adapt CACREP requirements. State licensing bodies accept applicants from academic programs that are not accredited by either CACREP or CORE, but these programs must be offered in academic institutions that are accredited by regional accrediting bodies and are recognized by the Department of Education (ACA, 2008b). Most states do not require that people graduate from counseling programs that specialize in mental health to become licensed as mental health counselors. Table 3.2 outlines the variation in training standards that are accepted by states for licensure of professional counselors.

### *Clinical and Face-to-Face Supervision Experience*

Clinical and face-to-face supervision experience varies widely among state licensure standards, as shown in Table 3.3. Requirements range from zero to 4,500 hours of supervised clinical experience and zero to 200 hours of face-to-face supervision.

**TABLE 3.2** State Educational and Clinical Practicum or Internship Requirements, 2009

| Training Standard | Required Educational Credits for Master's Degree | Required Clinical Practicum or Internship | No. States Using Standard[a] |
|---|---|---|---|
| Council for the Accreditation of Counseling and Related Educational Programs | • 48 semester hours<br>• 60 semester hours for mental health–counseling specialty | • 700 hours for standard counseling degree (no required experience in mental health setting)<br>• 1,000 hours for mental health–counseling specialty (including 360 direct service hours in mental health setting) | 18 |
| Commission on Rehabilitation Education | Master's in Rehabilitation Counseling | 700 hours (including 280 hours of direct service to people who have disabilities) | 2 |
| Regional or other state accreditation | Program-dependent; generally, 48–60 semester hours | Program-dependent; no specified standard for practicum or internship length unless specified by state | 10 |

*continued*

**TABLE 3.2** Continued

| Training Standard | Required Educational Credits for Master's Degree | Required Clinical Practicum or Internship | No. States Using Standard[a] |
|---|---|---|---|
| I. Master's in counseling<br>II. Graduate degree in allied mental health or related field<br>III. Graduate degree, including advanced counseling | • Program-dependent; 42–60 semester hours of graduate work, may include specific counseling coursework<br>• Some states permit "master's in a related field" with board determining whether program is equivalent to counseling; only specialty mental health–counseling programs require specific skill in diagnosis and treatment of persons who have mental disorders | Program-dependent; generally, internship of at least 600 hours; programs tend to gear requirements to ensure that graduates qualify to sit for credentialing examinations | 18 |

[a]Number of states that use the standard as their least rigorously defined requirement. Several states permit more than one education or training standard for licensure.
SOURCE: Adapted and updated from DOD (2006).

### *Examinations*

Licensing examinations vary by state, but the most common examinations required for licensure are the National Counselor Examination (NCE) and the National Clinical Mental Health Counselor Examination (NCMHCE)—both administered by NBCC—and the Certified Rehabilitation Counselor Examination (CRCE), administered by CORE. For their higher or highest level of licensure, 15 states and Puerto Rico require the NCE, 15 states require the NCMHCE,[2] 4 states require the NCE *and* NCMHCE, 7 states require either the NCE *or* the NCMHCE, 3 states require either the NCE or the CRCE, and 5 states

[2]One of these, Minnesota, requires the NCMHCE, but will alternatively accept the NCE and Examination of Clinical Counseling Practice, a discontinued NBCC examination.

**TABLE 3.3** State Requirements for Supervised Clinical Experience and Face-to-Face Supervision, 2009

| Supervised Clinical Experience | | Face-to-Face Supervision | |
|---|---|---|---|
| Hours | States | Hours | States |
| <2,000 | 2: ID, SC | None required | 26: AL, AR, AZ, CO, CT, DC, GA, IL, KS, MA, ME, MI, MN, MS, MT, NE, NJ, NY, OH, OR, PA, RI, TN, TX, WA, WV |
| 2,000–2,999 | 7: CO, GA, ME, MN, OR, RI, SD | 100 | 19: AK, DE, FL, HI, IA, IN, KY, LA, MD, NC, ND, NH, NM, NV, SC, SD, UT, VT, WY |
| 3,000–3,499 | 30: AK, AL, AR, AZ, CA, CT, DE, HI, IL, IN, LA, MA, MD, MI, MO, MT, ND, NE, NH, NV, NY, OH, OK, TN, TX, VT, WA, WI, WV, WY | 200 | 1: VA |
| 3,500–3,999 | 3: DC, MS, PA | 1–2 hours per week | 5: CA, ID, MO, OK, WI |
| >4,000 | 5: KS, KY, NJ, UT, VA | — | 0 |
| 2 years of post–master's degree supervised experience | 4: IA, FL, NC, NM | — | 0 |

SOURCE: Adapted and updated from DOD (2006).

and the District of Columbia accept any of the three examinations for licensure, as of late 2009.[3] Some states also allow additional or alternative examinations; others require additional examinations created by state licensing boards. Details regarding which states accept each examination are listed in Appendix G.

[3]California had yet to set its final examination requirements for licensure at the time this report was completed.

**The National Counselor Examination** The NCE is generic with respect to counseling. It covers the knowledge of counseling and counseling skills that should be known to all professional counselors regardless of field of practice. The NCE content outline has five content domains that consist of 130 tasks. The five domains and a sample of their tasks are listed in Table 3.4.

There are 200 multiple-choice items on the examination. They are based on the eight categories of core knowledge for professional counselors and the empirically determined five domains of professional-counselor work behaviors.

**The National Clinical Mental Health Counseling Examination** The NCMHCE is designed specifically for counselors who work in mental health. It is administered by NBCC.

The NCMHCE is a clinical-simulation examination that consists of 10 clinical mental health–counseling cases. Each case is divided into five to eight sections that are classified as information gathering or decision making. The cases cover the domains shown in Table 3.5.

A typical NCMHCE examination will include (NBCC, 2009d):

1. One simulation involving an adolescent client(s) with at least one primary clinical issue and at least one secondary clinical issue.
2. Three simulations with young adult clients with at least one primary clinical issue and at least one secondary clinical issue.
3. Four simulations with middle-aged clients with at least one primary clinical issue and at least one secondary clinical issue.
4. Two simulations with older adults clients with at least one primary clinical issue and at least one secondary clinical issue.

Primary clinical features on the examination would include such subjects as emotional abuse, suicidal issues, grief and loss, posttraumatic stress, depressive disorders, bipolar disorders, and adjustment disorders. Secondary clinical features would include such subjects as physical disabilities; homicidal, chronic medical, disaster-reaction, and substance-use–related issues; and schizophrenia and other psychoses, antisocial personality, and obsessive-compulsive disorder (NBCC, 2009c).

The committee notes that the use of simulations seems to be an appropriate strategy to test skills needed in a clinical mental health

**TABLE 3.4** National Counselor Examination Content Domains and Sample Tasks

| | |
|---|---|
| **I. Fundamentals of Counseling** | **III. Group Counseling** |
| 1. Assess client's progress toward counseling goals | 1. Facilitate group process |
| 2. Assess client's psychological functioning | 2. Assist group members in providing feedback to each other |
| 3. Conduct diagnostic interview | 3. Conduct postgroup follow-up procedures |
| 4. Assess need for client referral | 4. Identify behaviors that disrupt group process |
| 5. Diagnose on the basis of *DSM-IV-TR* criteria | 5. Assess progress toward group goals |
| **II. Assessment and Career Counseling** | **IV. Programmatic and Clinical Interventions** |
| 1. Use test results for client decision making | 1. Participate as member of multidisciplinary team |
| 2. Select and administer assessment instruments for counseling | 2. Provide crisis counseling to victims of disaster |
| 3. Provide career counseling for persons who have disabilities | 3. Assess programmatic needs |
| 4. Administer and interpret achievement tests | 4. Conduct community outreach |
| 5. Assess client's educational preparation | 5. Administer and manage counseling program |
| | **V. Professional-Practice Issues** |
| | 1. Evaluate the performance of other counselors |
| | 2. Provide diversity training |
| | 3. Provide clinical supervision for professionals |
| | 4. Engage in data analysis |
| | 5. Conduct community needs assessment |

SOURCE: NBCC (2009c).

practitioner, but it is not necessarily comprehensive enough to cover the breadth of diagnoses seen in the TRICARE system. It should be noted that the primary and secondary clinical features could lead to confusion if the *DSM-IV* is used for diagnosing purposes. Furthermore, although the content of the examination appears to be comprehensive, the use of such terms as *coordinate* and *function as a member of a multidisciplinary team/network* in the activities outline (NBCC, 2009c) content does not necessarily support independent practice. Task statements are not specific

**TABLE 3.5** National Clinical Mental Health Counseling Examination Case Domains and Sample Tasks

| Case Domain | Sample Items |
|---|---|
| **I. Evaluation and Assessment** | |
| • Identify precipitating problems or symptoms<br>• Conduct mental-status examination<br>• Identify individual and relationship functioning | • Conduct mental-status examination<br>—Cognitive functioning<br>—Affective functioning<br>—Suicidal and homicidal ideations<br>—Reality contact<br>—Alcohol and other drug use<br>• Conduct comprehensive biopsychosocial assessment histories<br>—Educational<br>—Addiction<br>—Sexual<br>—Psychiatric<br>—Trauma<br>—Psychiatric, medical, and addiction history of family system<br>—Current medications and diagnosed medical problems<br>• Interpret appraisal instruments and techniques<br>—Personality<br>—Intelligence |
| **II. Clinical Diagnosis and Treatment Planning** | |
| • Integrate client assessment and observational data with clinical judgment to formulate differential diagnosis<br>• Coordinate treatment plan with other service providers<br>• Monitor client progress toward goal attainment | • Formulate *DSM-IV* classification (axes I–V)<br>• Formulate *ICD-9-CM* classification<br>• Develop treatment plan in collaboration with client<br>• Establish goals that are relevant to diagnosis and client's needs<br>• Establish intervention strategies related to treatment objectives |

*continued*

**TABLE 3.5** Continued

| Case Domain | Sample Items |
|---|---|
| **III. Clinical Practice** | |
| • Determine whether services meet client's needs<br>• Understand scope of practice parameters<br>• Provide prevention interventions | • Implement counseling in relation to specific treatment plan<br>• Function as member of multidisciplinary team<br>• Educate client in need, effects, and impact of psychotropic medications<br>• Understand scope of practice parameters<br>—Liability issues<br>—Ethics |

Abbreviations: *DSM-IV* = *Diagnostic and Statistical Manual of Mental Disorders, 4th Edition, ICD-9-CM* = *International Classification of Diseases, 9th Revision, Clinical Modification.*
SOURCE: NBCC (2009c).

regarding testing for the ability to determine a "diagnosis" independently. *Treatment* is used in relation to "counseling" of a patient or client and not in a "medical model" sense of treatment for a diagnostic category. However, the term *counseling* appears to be used interchangeably with *psychotherapy* in the literature of the counseling profession.[4] In that sense, the use of *treatment* in relation to *counseling* would not be inconsistent. In addition, the terms *coordinate* and *function as a member of a multidisciplinary team/network* could also be interpreted as supporting the model of collaborative mental health care that is increasingly the standard of care in working with persons who have serious mental illness (Hoge et al., 2002). More specific task statements would be needed regarding specific treatment interventions to determine the body of knowledge that is being examined. The examination does seem to be aligned with the standard for an accredited academic program under CACREP.

Given those caveats, the NCMHCE's focus on clinical mental health counseling and on the evaluation of candidates' ability to apply knowledge to patient care led the committee to conclude that the examination is a more relevant test of the ability of counselors to serve

[4]In the mental health field, psychotherapy is generally defined as a practice that aims to remediate conflicts or symptoms related to psychopathology while facilitating growth. Counseling aims to enhance growth and facilitate adaptive functioning.

as independent providers of care than the NCEs. State licensure boards apparently share that view and use the NCMHCE as the examination applied to the more, or most rigorous, clinical level of licensure in many jurisdictions.

**The Certified Rehabilitation Counselor Examination** The CRCE is administered by CRCC (CRCC, 2009b). Requirements for sitting for the examination vary according to the applicant's level of education (master's versus doctoral degree) and the accreditation (if any) of the institution that granted the degree. They may include internship hours, employment experience, or specific coursework (CRCC, 2009a).

Twelve general knowledge domains underlie the examination. They are listed below, with additional detail in some aspects that are relevant to the practice of mental health counseling:

1. Career counseling and assessment.
2. Job development and placement services.
3. Vocational consultation and services for employers.
4. Case and caseload management.
5. Individual counseling, including individual counseling, behavior, and personality theories and multicultural counseling theories and practices.
6. Group and family counseling, including family and group counseling theories and multicultural counseling theories and practice.
7. Mental health counseling, including the *DSM*, rehabilitation techniques for individuals with psychiatric disabilities, multicultural counseling theories and practices, medications as they apply to individuals with psychiatric disabilities, dual diagnosis, substance abuse, treatment planning, and wellness and illness prevention concepts and strategies.
8. Psychosocial and cultural issues in counseling.
9. Medical, functional, and environmental aspects of disabilities, including medical aspects and implications of various disabilities, medications as they relate to vocational goals and outcomes, and functional capacities of individuals with physical, psychiatric, and/or cognitive disabilities.
10. Foundations, ethics, and professional issues.
11. Rehabilitation services and resources.

12. Health-care and disability systems, including managed-care concepts and insurance programs.

The test is administered electronically and comprises 150 scored and 25 field-test multiple-choice questions that span the domains listed above.

### *Ethical Standards*

Generally, the licensure of professionals has been presented to legislators and the general public in terms that make the argument that professional practitioners are skilled in assisting people in the fields of their expertise and must be granted licenses to protect the public from those who offer the same services without having specific training and credentials. Licensure boards adopt ethical and disciplinary standards and processes with the intent of ensuring competent practice. Thus, the ethical standards and disciplinary processes constitute the mechanisms through which incompetent or unethical practitioners will be regulated and removed from practice if their infractions are serious enough. Some questions have arisen concerning the degree to which professional licensure boards aggressively prosecute ethical infractions and whether individual practitioners do what they are licensed to do with competence and ethically (Corey et al., 2006; Duncan et al., 2004; Gross, 1979). The licensure mechanism is structured in such a manner that licensure boards adjudicate complaints brought to them and do not attempt to monitor the practices of behavioral health professionals to ensure the quality of care for clients. It is estimated that fewer than 1% of licensed counselors have ever been subjects of ethics complaints to state boards (Neukrug et al., 2001). That rate appears to be roughly the same as the rates reported by other professions. For example, the field of psychology experienced a rate of disciplinary complaints that was about 2% of licensed psychologists during 1996–2001 (Van Horne, 2004). Despite the concerns raised, licensure boards constitute a powerful part of the credentialing system and prevent harmful or unethical practitioners from continuing in practice in their jurisdictions.

In general, licensure boards adopt in whole or in part the codes of ethics of the professional discipline they are related to, which typically are set forth by the major professional associations. Beyond that, other standards in administrative rules may supplement those ethical codes, such as the requirement to pay annual licensing fees in a timely manner. Apart from administrative rules, sexual misconduct with clients is thought to be so serious that it is subject to criminal legal sanctions in an increasing number of states, including California, Colorado, Florida, Georgia, Idaho, Maine, Michigan, Minnesota, Washington, and Wisconsin. Other states are working toward passage of such legislation to supplant licensure boards' governance related to this most serious of ethical infractions (Reaves, 2003).

The profession of licensed mental health counseling has followed the same general pattern as the other behavioral health disciplines. ACA reports that as of December 2009, 17 jurisdictions had adopted the ACA Code of Ethics into their rules and regulations: Alaska, Arizona, Arkansas, District of Columbia, Idaho, Illinois, Iowa, Louisiana, Massachusetts, Mississippi, North Carolina, North Dakota, South Dakota, Tennessee, Utah, West Virginia, and Wyoming (ACA, 2010). It notes that three states (Colorado, Ohio, and South Carolina) refer to the ACA code for advice on ethical guidelines or to use as an aid in resolving ambiguities in disciplinary rules. Delaware has adopted the NBCC Code of Ethics (State of Delaware, 2010). Some other states—Minnesota, for example—enforce their own codes of ethics (Minnesota Administrative Rules 2150.7500 *CONDUCT*).

The ACA code has a number of strictures regarding counselors' ethical obligations to provide services only within their competence and scope of practice, to diagnose properly, to educate themselves in and apply scientifically based treatment modalities, and to appropriately refer patients who present with problems outside their competence and scope of practice. Relevant clauses are listed in Table 3.6. NBCC has similar requirements.

A nonscientific, annual survey of its member licensure boards conducted by the American Association of State Counseling Boards documents that ethical standards are being used by licensure boards to discipline their licensees (AASCB, 2008). For 2008, the survey of member boards reported that 395 licensees were disciplined in connection with 1,065 complaints received in the 27 states that reported data. There were a total of 81,309 licensees in the reporting jurisdictions. The 1.3% complaint rate in this informal survey is consistent with the rates of complaints to licensure boards reported in the literature. Among the 395 licensees disciplined, there were 33 revocations, 33 suspensions, 83 disciplinary letters, 3 criminal prosecutions, and 305 other actions reported.

**TABLE 3.6** Excerpts from ACA Code of Ethics Related to Professional Competence

**A.11. Termination and Referral**
**A.11.b. Inability to Assist Clients**
If counselors determine an inability to be of professional assistance to clients, they avoid entering or continuing counseling relationships. Counselors are knowledgeable about culturally and clinically appropriate referral resources and suggest these alternatives. If clients decline the suggested referrals, counselors should discontinue the relationship.

**A.11.c. Appropriate Termination**
Counselors terminate a counseling relationship when it becomes reasonably apparent that the client no longer needs assistance, is not likely to benefit, or is being harmed by continued counseling....

**C.2. Professional Competence**
**C.2.a. Boundaries of Competence**
Counselors practice only within the boundaries of their competence, based on their education, training, supervised experience, state and national professional credentials, and appropriate professional experience. Counselors gain knowledge, personal awareness, sensitivity, and skills pertinent to working with a diverse client population.

**C.2.b. New Specialty Areas of Practice**
Counselors practice in specialty areas new to them only after appropriate education, training, and supervised experience. While developing skills in new specialty areas, counselors take steps to ensure the competence of their work and to protect others from possible harm.

**C.2.c. Qualified for Employment**
Counselors accept employment only for positions for which they are qualified by education, training, supervised experience, state and national professional credentials, and appropriate professional experience. Counselors hire for professional counseling positions only individuals who are qualified and competent for those positions.

**C.2.d. Monitor Effectiveness**
Counselors continually monitor their effectiveness as professionals and take steps to improve when necessary. Counselors in private practice take reasonable steps to seek peer supervision as needed to evaluate their efficacy as counselors.

**C.2.f. Continuing Education**
Counselors recognize the need for continuing education to acquire and maintain a reasonable level of awareness of current scientific and professional information in their fields of activity. They take steps to maintain competence in the skills they use, are open to new procedures, and keep current with the diverse populations and specific populations with whom they work.

*continued*

**TABLE 3.6** Continued

| |
|---|
| **C.6.e. Scientific Bases for Treatment Modalities**<br>Counselors use techniques/procedures/modalities that are grounded in theory and/or have an empirical or scientific foundation. Counselors who do not must define the techniques/procedures as "unproven" or "developing" and explain the potential risks and ethical considerations of using such techniques/procedures and take steps to protect clients from possible harm. |
| **D.1.c. Interdisciplinary Teamwork**<br>Counselors who are members of interdisciplinary teams delivering multifaceted services to clients keep the focus on how to best serve the clients. They participate in and contribute to decisions that affect the well-being of clients by drawing on the perspectives, values, and experiences of the counseling profession and those of colleagues from other disciplines. |
| **D.2.a. Consultant Competency**<br>Counselors take reasonable steps to ensure that they have the appropriate resources and competencies when providing consultation services. Counselors provide appropriate referral resources when requested or needed. |
| **E.5. Diagnosis of Mental Disorders**<br>**E.2.a. Limits of Competence**<br>Counselors utilize only those testing and assessment services for which they have been trained and are competent. Counselors using technology-assisted test interpretations are trained in the construct being measured and the specific instrument being used prior to using its technology-based application. Counselors take reasonable measures to ensure the proper use of psychological and career assessment techniques by persons under their supervision. |
| **E.5.a. Proper Diagnosis**<br>Counselors take special care to provide proper diagnosis of mental disorders. Assessment techniques (including personal interview) used to determine client care (e.g., locus of treatment, type of treatment, or recommended follow-up) are carefully selected and appropriately used. |
| **F.2. Counselor Supervision Competence**<br>**F.2.a. Supervisor Preparation**<br>Prior to offering clinical supervision services, counselors are trained in supervision methods and techniques. Counselors who offer clinical supervision services regularly pursue continuing education activities including both counseling and supervision topics and skills. |

SOURCE: ACA (2005).

Adherence to such codes helps to ensure that practitioners provide services within their expertise and results in specific disciplinary actions by counseling licensure boards that protect the public.

### Criteria for Maintaining Licensure

Criteria for maintaining licensure vary but may include continuing education hours and maintenance of a "clean" record of adherence to ethical standards or other standards of professional or personal conduct.

The number of required continuing education hours for maintaining licensure varies by state from zero to 55 hours every 2 years. Licensure renewal is required by all states; the frequency of renewal ranges from once a year to once every 3 years. A complete list of continuing education and license renewal requirements is provided in Appendix G.

## CERTIFICATION BY STANDARDS ASSOCIATIONS

Licensure and certification are viewed as complementary mechanisms; certification is thought to help in standardizing licensure requirements across states in that national certification examinations are often used as prerequisites for licensure. In the field of counseling, both require master's level or higher degrees, a practicum or internship experience, supervised counseling experience, direct supervision, and passage of a counselor examination administered at the state or national level (Clawson, 2009).

Voluntary professional certification involves a systematic process and action by a duly authorized independent third party that determines, verifies, and attests in writing to the competences of people in a profession in accordance with applicable requirements associated with that profession. Major components of a certification process typically include the following:

- A specified scope of the certification.
- A well-defined code of ethics.
- A job or practice analysis to identify competencies.

- Translation of the results of the job or practice analysis into a test blueprint that includes knowledge statements and task statements.
- Examinations that are constructed to have psychometric rigor of fairness, validity, and reliability.
- Scientific methods to determine the passing score.
- A recertification program that demonstrates continued competence.
- Processes to remove certification from a person.

The organization responsible for certifying mental health counselors at the national level is NBCC. CRCC performs an analogous function for rehabilitation counselors. The certifications granted by those organizations are discussed in the following sections. Other counseling specialties have their own governing bodies and certifications.

### National Certified Counselor Certification

NBCC is an independent not-for-profit credentialing body for counselors. It was incorporated in 1982 to establish and monitor a national certification system, identify counselors who have sought and obtained certification, and maintain a register of certified counselors (NBCC, 2009a). NBCC's primary focus is on promoting high-quality counseling. National certification by NBCC is a voluntary extra step taken by professionals in addition to required state counselor credentialing.

The basic educational requirements for the national certified counselor (NCC) credential are based on the CACREP accreditation standards and include a master's degree in a counseling-related field from a regionally accredited institution, 48 semester hours of graduate study in the practice of counseling and closely related fields, and a counseling course in each of eight content categories. The categories are human growth and development, social and cultural foundations, helping relationships, group work, career and lifestyle development, appraisal, research and program evaluation, and professional orientation and ethics. In addition to those educational requirements, required clinical experience includes two academic terms of graduate-level, supervised field experience in a counseling setting; 2 years of post-master's counseling experience (not necessary if the counselor graduated from a CACREP-accredited institution), 3,000 hours of client contact and 100 hours of face-to-face supervision, and passage of the NCE (NBCC, 2010).

### Certified Clinical Mental Health Counselor Certification

The Certified Clinical Mental Health Counselor (CCMHC) certification was launched in 1979 under the National Academy for Certified Clinical Mental Health Counselors (NACCMHC), an organization formed by the American Mental Health Counselors Association. In 1993, NACCMHC and NBCC came to an agreement whereby NBCC would administer the CCMHC credential beginning July 1, 1993. The credential is sometimes used as an alternative method for meeting the requirements for becoming licensed in a state and may be one of the requirements for independent practice in a state.

Certification eligibility requirements are (NBCC, 2009b)

- The NCC credential.
- A passing score on the NCMHCE.
- 60 semester hours or 90 quarter hours of graduate coursework, including a separate course of at least 2 semester hours or 3 quarter hours in
  - —Theories of counseling psychotherapy and personality, including studies of basic theories, principles and techniques of counseling, and their application to professional counseling settings.
  - —Counseling and psychotherapy skills, including training in basic counseling skills, consultation, and crisis intervention.
  - —Abnormal psychotherapy and psychopathology, including training in diagnosis (*DSM-III-R* or *DSM-IV*), psychopharmacology, and treatment methods for mental and emotional disorders.
  - —Human growth and development.
  - —Group counseling and psychotherapy, including coursework in group dynamics and development, group counseling and psychotherapy theory, and group methods and techniques.
  - —Career development.
  - —Professional orientation to counseling.
  - —Research.

—Testing and appraisal, including individual and group approaches to assessment and evaluation and interview assessment procedures.
—Social and cultural foundations.

- Clinical training:
  —9–15 semester hours or 14–23 quarter hours.
  —Counseling supervisors must have at least a master's degree in an allied mental health field and 5 years of post-master's work experience or a doctorate in an allied mental health field and 3 years of postdoctoral work experience. (Additional requirements are also imposed on supervisors.)

The committee notes that the diversity of academic preparation and clinical internship experiences among the different types of approved supervision may lead to different outcomes. That may raise concern about the consistency and standardization that are needed to ensure common outcomes of students among academic programs or even within an academic program. Again, however, it is a generic issue and not one peculiar to mental health–counseling certifications.

## Certified Rehabilitation Counselor Certification

The Certified Rehabilitation Counselor credential is administered by CRCC (CRCC, 2009b). Certification is granted on successful completion of the CRCE. CRCC requires that counselors renew their certification every 5 years by documenting the accrual of at least 100 clock hours of continuing education or by reexamination. Certificants are also obliged to conform to the commission's Code of Professional Ethics for Rehabilitation Counselors as overseen by an ethics committee.

This certification is recognized by the National Commission for Certifying Agencies. Nine states require the CRCE to become licensed as a professional counselor (ACA, 2008b). The 12 general knowledge domains that underlie the CRCE are listed above.

## RECOGNITION OF THIRD-PARTY CERTIFICATIONS BY THE DEPARTMENT OF DEFENSE

The committee's statement of task called for it to examine Department of Defense (DOD) recognition of third-party certification for members of the mental health professions. The department routinely relies on such certification on the basis of authority in the *Code of Federal Regulations.* Title 32 of Section 199.6 (excerpted in Appendix D) states that clinical psychologists, certified clinical social workers, certified psychiatric nurse specialists, certified marriage and family therapists, pastoral counselors, and mental health counselors must be licensed or certified by the jurisdiction where they wish to practice. For jurisdictions that do not offer licensure or certification, providers must be "certified by or eligible for full clinical membership in the appropriate national professional association that sets standards for the specific profession." For counselors, the *TRICARE Policy Manual* (6010.54-M, Chapter 11, Section 3.10) sets the following standard:

> In jurisdictions that do not offer licensure, the mental health counselor must be (or must meet all of the requirements to become) a Certified Clinical Mental Health Counselor (CCMHC) as determined by the Clinical Academy of the National Board of Certified Counselors (NBCC).

Other organizations recognized by TRICARE for certification of practitioners or their educational institutions include the National Register of Health Service Providers in Psychology for clinical psychologists, the CSWE for certified clinical social workers, and the American Association of Pastor Counselors.

A "qualified accreditation organization" is defined in 32 CFR § 199.2 as a not-for-profit corporation or foundation that develops knowledge and skill standards for health-care–professional certification testing, creates measurable criteria, publishes the standards and evaluation processes, provides national testing of people, provides written certification of compliance to people, publishes the outcomes for the general public, and "has been found by the Director, OCHAMPUS, or designee, to apply standards, criteria, and certification processes which reinforce CHAMPUS provider authorization requirements and promote efficient delivery of CHAMPUS benefits."

## CREDENTIALING AND PRIVILEGING

Health-care organizations (HCOs) ensure high-quality health care for their beneficiaries in part by ascertaining that their health-care providers meet established professional standards of education, training, and ethical conduct as demonstrated and validated by appropriate diplomas, licenses, and certificates. Credentialing involves the review and usually primary source verification of each practitioner's professional document portfolio. Privileging—the authorization of a variety, scope, and content of professional activities for each practitioner by an HCO—is based not only on careful review and evaluation of each practitioner's credentials and performance but on the mission, scope, and specific needs of the organization.

In the TRICARE system, both the direct-care system (military health-care facilities) and the contracted-out (purchased-care) system have specific credentialing and privileging requirements. These and practices in the private sector are discussed below.

### Credentialing and Privileging in TRICARE

#### *TRICARE Direct-Care System*

**Overview** Credentialing and privileging requirements in the direct-care system are outlined in the appropriate service regulations or instructions, specifically Army Regulation 40-68; Navy BUMEDINST 6320.66E; and Air Force Instruction 44-119. The policies apply not only to active-duty people and others employed by each service but to other providers (e.g., volunteers and members of other services) who are not classified as employees of the particular service but are providing patient care under the auspices of the military or based on guidelines articulated in a US or foreign memoranda of understanding or memoranda of agreement.[5]

Credentialing and privileging policies are the responsibility of each service's medical department, ultimately the service's surgeon general. Specific privileges of each credentialed practitioner are delineated in each clinical department by the appropriate department chief; this

[5]A memorandum of understanding or memorandum of agreement would be used, for example, for non-US health-care personnel deployed in a theater of operations.

delineation must be approved by the medical treatment facility (MTF) commander—or, in the Navy, by a higher headquarters commander—who is the sole approval authority for each MTF in the Military Health System.

Providers are granted only clinical privileges that are appropriate for the settings in which they practice. A cardiothoracic surgeon practicing in an outpatient cardiology clinic, for example, will not be granted privileges to perform bypass surgery in the clinic; and a psychiatrist trained in electroconvulsive therapy (ECT) will not be granted privileges to perform ECT in a community mental health facility that is not equipped or staffed to support the procedure.

US Army, Navy, and Air Force requirements relevant to mental health–care providers are outlined below.

**Army** Army Regulation 40–68—*Clinical Quality Management*—delineates the service's general policies on licensure, certification, and registration of health-care professionals. Appendix E excerpts several sections of the regulation that are relevant to the discussion below.

Section 4-4 of Regulation 40–68 provides a "not all inclusive" list of the professional disciplines requiring license, certification, or registration to practice in the Army. The list specifically mentions clinical psychologists, clinical social workers, counseling psychologists, physicians, psychological associates, substance-abuse counselors, and "behavioral health practitioners."

Guidance regarding the scope of practice and other specific professional requirements for privileged providers is in Section 7. Section 7-6 addresses "behavioral health practitioners." These are defined as persons who "are trained in behavioral science, counseling theories, and practical applications of behavior change principles" and "may manage numerous behavioral and emotional problems, in both general and particular specialty practice levels, providing a variety of behavioral health services, including screening, treatment, and consultation." The regulation adds that "the behavioral health practitioner may develop additional expertise in psychometrics, industrial psychology, substance abuse rehabilitation, geriatric care, school or health psychology, neuropsychology, pediatric or adolescent psychology, aeromedical psychology, and combat stress reactions."

Section 7-6b describes a three-tier privileging system for behavioral health practitioners. A Category I practitioner "performs specialty counseling services and works under the supervision of a psychologist, psychiatrist, or clinical social worker licensed in his/her discipline" and is required to have a master's degree in counseling psychology, including "a minimum of 12 supervised practicum hours in the major specialty" and "either the Licensed Professional Counselor (LPC) license or a master's level psychology license, such as psychological associate license, from a State licensing board." The regulation notes that "some States use a different title for their LPC-equivalent license" and "the education and experience requirements for licensure are the basis for determining equivalency." Category II requires in addition "a minimum of 2 years' full-time experience in the specialty in which services are performed under the supervision of a higher level privileged provider with a license in social work, psychology, or psychiatry." Category III is for practitioners who provide "a wide range of services in the designated specialty and may supervise category II or I counselors in their provision of services in the specialty" but still need to "be supervised by a psychologist, psychiatrist, or a social worker who is licensed in their respective disciplines and privileged at a higher level (category)."

Section 7-6c states that practitioners will "practice within the guidelines of their respective State licensing boards as LPCs (or equivalent) or, if offered by their State, a license for master's-level psychology graduates such as psychological associate or licensed mental health provider." Specific clinical privileges are "granted based upon training, experience, and competency." Five general privileges are delineated:

1. Conduct screening evaluations, utilizing information from clinical interviews, nonpsychometric tests, and collateral sources, as appropriate.
2. Determine a provisional diagnosis according to the American Psychiatric Association *Diagnostic and Statistical Manual of Mental Disorders.*
3. Provide individual and group behavioral health treatment within the scope of practice/privileges granted.
4. Manage the behavioral health care of patients and refer those having needs beyond their scope of practice.
5. Serve as collaborator in human behavioral issues with, and consultant to, community agencies, health care providers, and organizational leaders.

Two companion forms are used to document the delineation and evaluation of clinical privileges for behavioral health practitioners for specific providers: Department of the Army (DA) Forms 5440-34 and 5441-34. These include checkoffs for various types of assessment (psychological, substance abuse, adult, adolescent, and family), treatment planning (inpatient and outpatient), and categories of patients and therapy (adult, adolescent, family, marital, individual, group, crisis, inpatient, and outpatient). No specific therapies are listed, but the delineation of clinical privileges for "substance abuse rehabilitation"[6] (DA Form 5440–58) offers insight into how this is accomplished in the Army. The form lists eight kinds of therapy for which practice privileges may be requested and approved (cognitive-behavioral and rational-emotive, reality, brief, gestalt, psychodynamic, group, and transactional analysis) with blanks for additions.

**Navy** General Navy and Marine Corps policies on licensure, certification, and registration of health-care professionals are articulated in Bureau of Medicine and Surgery Instruction (BUMEDINST) 6320.66E, *Credentials Review and Privileging Program.* They are quite similar to the Army instructions reviewed above except that in the latest ("E" ) version of Instruction 6320.66, authority for privileging providers in fixed medical and dental facilities is delegated by the chief of BUMED to higher headquarters commanders (medical regional commanders) rather than to facility commanders directly. Guidelines for clinical privileging and credentials review of "Clinical Practitioners/Providers in Department of the Navy Fleet and Family Support Program and Marine Corps Community Services" are provided in SECNAV Instruction 1754.7 (November 2005).

Section 8a(2), BUMEDINST 6320.66E, states that "Chief, BUMED shall: Establish, in coordination with chiefs of the appropriate corps and the specialty leaders, standardized clinical privilege sheets, which prescribe both core and supplemental privileges reflecting the currently recognized scope of care for each health care specialty." Section 10d adds:

---

[6]Professionals who practice substance-abuse rehabilitation have educational and licensing requirements similar to those of behavioral health practitioners.

> Privileging authorities shall grant clinical privileges to health care practitioners using standardized, specialty specific privilege sheets contained in this instruction. These privilege sheets reflect the currently recognized scope of care appropriate to each health care specialty. Commanding officers shall ensure health care practitioners provide care consistent with their approved clinical privileges.

Appendix G (pages G-1–G-38) of BUMEDINST 6320.66E contains clinical-privilege sheets for the allied-health professions and outlines the educational requirements for each specialty. Clinical psychologists, clinical social workers, and marriage and family therapists are all addressed, but behavioral health practitioners and mental health counselors are not mentioned on this list or elsewhere in the instruction. A reasonable inference is that licensed counselors are not used in Navy health care facilities.

Counselors are, however, used in the Navy Fleet and Family Support Program (FFSP) and Marine Corps Community Services (MCCS) as documented in SECNAV Instruction 1754.7. The procedures outlined in the instruction are similar to those in other military facilities. Section 9a(1) states that "clinical practitioners include, but are not limited to, privileged psychologists, social workers, and marriage and family therapists"; and the instruction focuses on these behavioral health providers.

SECNAV Instruction 1754.7A, *Process of Credentials Review and Privileging,* sets up a three-tier privileging system similar to the Army's. Tier I "includes entry-level providers who are collecting their supervised clinical hours to be applied toward licensure" and who are expected to complete their licensure/certification within a 36-month period. Tier II "includes providers who are State licensed or State certified or were granted a license or a certificate by a U.S. territory to provide independent clinical care." Tier III "includes providers who are State licensed or State certified or were granted a license or a certificate by a U.S. territory, have been granted clinical privileges to function as an independent practitioner, and have attained specified additional clinical experience."

Section 3 of SECNAV Instruction 1754.7A, which addresses the "minimum qualifications and capabilities of providers functioning within this three-tier system," lists a master's or doctoral degree in counseling from a program accredited by CACREP or an equivalent degree as meeting the requirement for Tier I privileging only. In addition to other requirements, providers privileged at Tier II or III are required to have at least a master's degree in marital and family therapy, psychology, or social work. Similarly, the list of core privileges provided in Enclosure 3 addresses privileges for those three disciplines but does not mention counselors. A reasonable conclusion is that the Navy uses counselors in the FFSP and MCCS but privileges them only at the Tier I level.

**Air Force** General policies on licensure, certification, and registration of health-care professionals are articulated in Chapters 4, 5, and 6 of Air Force Instruction 44-119, *Medical Quality Operations*. These are consistent with and similar to those in the Army and the Navy. Section 5.3 refers to the Centralized Credentials and Quality Assurance System (CCQAS), a DOD-mandated Web-based secure credentials and risk-management application used in the provider credentialing and privileging process, and it lists the categories of providers that according to DOD must be included in CCQAS. The list is similar to that of allied health professions included in Appendix G of Navy BUMEDINST 6320.66E in that it lists clinical psychologists, marriage and family therapists, and social workers; but it also mentions mental health counselors (to include certified alcohol and drug-abuse counselors) and professional counselors.

Chapter 7 of the instruction addresses the professional scope of practice for allied health. Section 7A presents an allied health provider list. It includes psychiatric and mental health nurse practitioners, psychologists, and social workers but does not mention mental health or other counselors or marriage and family therapists. Another list, "non-privileged Allied Health Professionals," in Section 7B, specifically mentions certified alcohol and drug-abuse counselors. This suggests that, although counselors are mentioned in the categories of providers that are to be included in CCQAS if used by the services, they are probably not currently used by the Air Force.

### *TRICARE Purchased-Care System*

As mentioned in Chapter 1, the purchased-care contractors in 2009 were MHN/HealthNet for TRICARE North, Humana for TRICARE South, and TriWest for TRICARE West. In July 2009, it was announced that new contracts had been awarded to Aetna Government Health

Plans for the north region, UnitedHealth Military & Veterans Services for the south region, and TriWest for the west region. The information below addresses the contractors serving in 2009.

Purchased-care contractors must conform to the policies articulated in *TRICARE Policy Manual* 6010.54 (August 2002). Although policies dictate that counselors be credentialed, the details are left to the contractor. In a presentation to the committee in July 2009, a representative of MHN/HealthNet indicated that the following criteria—which largely overlap the regulatory requirements—were applied by his firm (Shaffer, 2009):

- A degree from a US professional school that includes education and training commensurate with state requirements for licensure. A waiver can be applied for if the applicant graduated from a non-US school.
- A current, independent license or certification in the state where practice will occur.
- Professional liability insurance $1 million per occurrence/ $1 million aggregate, with lower limits possible when such are the community standard or when the MHN level of insurance is not available.
- Two years of post-master's experience which includes 3,000 hours of clinical work and 100 hours of face-to-face supervision.

MHN/HealthNet's credentialing application process included primary source verification of education, license, and insurance; a review of the applicant's history of insurance actions and license investigations; and a criminal-background check. That information needed to be examined and approved by the Credential Committee before a contract with the applicant was completed. MHN/HealthNet did not engage in case-specific or treatment-specific privileging but did ask providers to identify subjects of specific expertise in client subpopulations (children and adolescents, for example), in diagnosis, and in treatment modalities (such as dialectical behavioral therapy) (Shaffer, 2009).

TriWest provides specific credentialing forms for each behavioral discipline; the form for counselors conforms to TRICARE requirements regarding referral and supervision by a physician. Humana's *Provider Handbook* does not address privileging and scope of practice beyond claim and billing considerations.

The committee did not identify any circumstance in which the contractor defined the scope of practice for any particular discipline beyond the boundaries prescribed by each practitioner's professional license and in anything other than general terms.

Supervisory policies are similarly vague. MHN/HealthNet indicated that it does not set specific criteria for the form and manner of physicians' supervision of counselors beyond that specified in 32 CFR § 199.6 (Appendix D). Physicians are simply reminded that they have a responsibility to supervise (Shaffer, 2009).

## Private Sector

Provider credentialing in private-sector HCOs is heavily shaped by the accreditation standards established by the National Committee for Quality Assurance (NCQA) and URAC.[7] All contracted providers must be credentialed and, for most managed-care behavioral health organizations (MBHOs), must be licensed. Accreditation standards require MBHOs to verify from the primary source (directly contacting the source that has issued the training, certification, and so on) the training, licensure, certification, malpractice filing history (only available for MDs), report of "good standing" in the community (absence of an important criminal record or complaints to licensing boards and existence of references from colleagues) of each independent practitioner. MBHOs also collect signed attestation statements at the time of credentialing and recredentialing to disclose any criminal action, substance abuse, or mental impairment. Providers who practice in clinics or facilities that are not accredited are treated and must be credentialed as independent providers. Providers who practice in facilities or clinics that are accredited—by the Joint Commission or the Commission on Accreditation of Rehabilitation Facilities (CARF)—are credentialed by hiring entities that follow the standards of the Joint Commission and CARF. MBHOs have the option to accept an accredited clinic or facility credentialing process and not duplicate the process. MBHOs are required to recredential providers every 3 years, updating such information as licensure status, attestations, complaints, sentinel events, and, in some MBHOs, patient satisfaction.

---

[7]URAC is the formal name of the accreditation organization originally incorporated as the Utilization Review Accreditation Commission (URAC, 2009).

Other than conforming to state law, there is no consistent pattern or single set of rules applied to determine whether or under what circumstances a particular class of providers may have their services eligible for reimbursement or subject to referral or supervision requirements. Indeed, a class of providers that may be covered under one plan offered by an insurer might not be covered under a different plan offered by the same insurer. Decisions in such cases are driven by cost considerations and by the preferences of the organization that contracts with the insurer. For example, a religious organization may require that its plan cover the services of pastoral counselors.

The scope of practice for all contracted providers is dictated by their professional licensure, certifications where they exist, fellowships, and special training. Scopes of practice linked to formal certifications or fellowships are verified and included in the scopes of practice of a provider. Most behavioral health diagnoses and treatments do not have recognized designations of competency that are consistent and reliable, such as board certifications or subspecialty fellowships that are accredited. Complex conditions, such as eating disorders and traumatic brain injury, that require expertise do not have recognized certifications or accredited fellowships.

In the absence of those formal designations, other forms of information are collected by self-reporting to identify providers who have experience or expertise, such as the percentage of practice devoted to a specific diagnostic category or population type and postgraduate continuing education courses. In many MBHOs, providers are given a list of diagnoses and evidence-based treatments at the time of credentialing and recredentialing and are asked to indicate the scope of diagnosis and treatment in which they have experience or expertise.

Communication of provider expertise to patients is not addressed by accreditation standards. There is great variability in how providers' experience is communicated when patients are selecting providers. All MBHOs list providers' professional training credentials (such as MD, PhD, LPC, MFT, and CSW) and certifications. Beyond those designations, self-reported experience varies. CIGNA HealthCare, for example, displays on its Web site not only a provider's credentials and experience but a photograph (if submitted by the provider) and a brief paragraph written by the provider to give a more personal introduction and description of her or his fields of practice and clinical approach.

Monitoring of the performance of independent providers, facilities, and clinics in the network of an MBHO generally follows accreditation standards. The standard monitoring touch points are as follows:

- Patient safety (all items are recorded by individual provider, facility, or clinic):
  - —Complaints registered with the MBHO (ongoing and real-time review).
  - —Reported sentinel events such as suicide and assault (ongoing and real-time review).
  - —Complaints collected through licensing board (every 3 years).
  - —Site-visit review of environment and office procedures (record storage, onsite medication storage, and the like) (randomly selected or focused on high-volume providers).
- Quality reporting:
  - —Compliance with practice guidelines.
  - —Patient satisfaction.
  - —Utilization patterns.
  - —Standardized Healthcare Effectiveness Data and Information Set (HEDIS)[8] performance measures:
    - Measurement of postdischarge outpatient care.
    - Measurement of antidepressant-medication management for depression.
    - Measurement of ADHD-medication management.
    - Measurement of alcohol-use and substance-use screening and treatment engagement.
  - —Other nonstandard measurements as designated by the MBHO.

Patient-safety data collection and review is ongoing for complaints and sentinel events reported to the MBHO. The MBHO must investigate, review, and resolve all complaints and sentinel events typically within 30 days. Members involved in the complaints and sentinel events are notified of the outcomes when that is appropriate. When unsafe practices are identified, the MBHO takes action with the provider, facil-

[8]HEDIS is a tool administered by NCQA and "used by more than 90 percent of America's health plans to measure performance on important dimensions of care and service" (NCQA, 2009).

ity, or clinic. Typical actions include creation of corrective-action plans with oversight until conclusion, removal from the network, and reporting to licensing and certification boards or accreditation bodies.

Most quality reporting is at the institutional level; it is seldom by individual providers. Resource limitations, technology limitations, and insufficient volume for an accurate measurement are the major factors that keep MBHOs from reporting on a provider level. Because MBHOs have such large networks and providers are selected by patients, it is difficult to accumulate a sufficient volume of patients being treated by a specific provider and belonging to the MBHO. Most MBHOs, if provider-level performance measures are collected and reported, focus on high-volume providers (generally 10–15 patients per provider during the measurement period) to obtain results that have a degree of validity.

Monitoring of compliance with stated scopes of practice by providers, including licensed counselors is not done in a formal or direct way in MBHOs. The lack of clear designation of scope of practice from subspecialty training programs and the lack of national criteria for setting standards for designating scope of practice pose a problem in determining with any validity a provider's scope of practice beyond certifications and self-reporting. Technology and data-collection systems required to address that task would be expensive and labor-intensive. If there are complaints and sentinel events regarding the quality of service of specific providers, MBHOs review patient-safety trends at the time of recredentialing or each time an event is reported. During the investigation of a complaint or sentinel event, whatever scope-of-practice issues arise are addressed.

Some MBHOs have initiated the measurement of treatment outcomes for their providers. For example, OptumHealth Behavioral Solutions (OHBS)—through its ALERT program—requires the use of a valid global distress measurement for adults and children at baseline and during therapy by all contracted providers. The trend of outcome measurements is observed for high-volume providers (10 or more patients each with two data points), effect size and (a benchmarked measurement of clinical effectiveness) is reported. OHBS has started to tier providers on the basis of their scores—specifically, the ability to achieve clinical effectiveness with all their OHBS patients—and to make the tiering status available to members who seek care.

**BOX 3.1**
**Abbreviations and Acronyms**

**Accrediting bodies and professional associations**

| | |
|---|---|
| ACA | American Counseling Association |
| ACGME | Accreditation Council for Graduate Medical Education |
| AMHCA | American Mental Health Counselors Association |
| APA | American Psychological Association |
| APA CoA | APA Commission on Accreditation |
| CACREP | Council for Accreditation of Counseling and Related Educational Programs |
| CARF | Commission on Accreditation of Rehabilitation Facilities |
| CCNE | Commission on Collegiate Nursing Education |
| CHEA | Council on Higher Education Accreditation |
| CORE | Council on Rehabilitation Education |
| CRCC | Commission on Rehabilitation Counselor Certification |
| CSWE | Council on Social Work Education |
| LCME | Liaison Committee on Medical Education |
| NACCMHC | National Academy for Certified Clinical Mental Health Counselors |
| NBCC | National Board for Certified Counselors |
| NCCA | National Commission for Certifying Agencies |
| NCQA | National Committee for Quality Assurance |
| The Joint Commission | *formerly, the Joint Commission on Accreditation of Healthcare Organizations (JCAHO)* |
| URAC | *the current name of the organization originally incorporated as the "Utilization Review Accreditation Commission"* |

**Certifications in the field of counseling**

| | |
|---|---|
| CCMHC | Certified Clinical Mental Health Counselor |
| CRC | Certified Rehabilitation Counselor |
| NCC | National Certified Counselor |

**Counseling examinations**

| | |
|---|---|
| CRCE | Certified Rehabilitation Counselor Examination |
| NCE | National Counselor Examination |
| NCMHCE | National Clinical Mental Health Counselor Examination |

# REFERENCES

AAMFT (American Association for Marriage and Family Therapy). 2004. *Marriage and Family Therapy core competencies, December.* http://www.antiochne.edu/AP/mftphd/AAMFTCoreComptencies.pdf. (Accessed November 7, 2009).

AAPC (American Association of Pastoral Counselors). 2009. *About pastoral counseling.* http://www.aapc.org/content/about-pastoral-counseling. (Accessed November 7, 2009).

AASCB (American Association of State Counseling Boards). 2008. *Summary of 2008 state licensing board reports.* http://www.aascb.org/associations/7905/files/State_Board_Report_Summary_2008.pdf. (Accessed October 12, 2009).

ACA (American Counseling Association). 2005. *Code of ethics.* Washington, DC: American Counseling Association.

ACA. 2008. *Licensure requirements for professional counselors: A state-by-state report.* Alexandria, VA: ACA.

ACA. 2010. *State licensure boards that have adopted the ACA Code of Ethics—2010.* http://www.counseling.org/Files/FD.ashx?guid=1bf2d9ae-6c26-412b-b123-147991e59350. (Accessed January 7, 2010).

ACGME (Accreditation Council for Graduate Medical Education). 2007. Accreditation Council for Graduate Medical Education. http://www.acgme.org. (Accessed November 7, 2009).

Altekruse MK, Harris HL, Brandt MA. 2001. The role of the professional counselor in the 21st century. *Counseling and Human Development* 34:1-10.

APA CoA (American Psychological Association Commission on Accreditation). 2008. *Guidelines and principles for accreditation of programs in professional psychology.* http://www.apa.org/ed/accreditation/G&P0522.pdf. (Accessed June 22, 2009).

Benjamin LT Jr. 2006. *A history of psychology in letters,* 2nd ed. Chichester, England: Blackwell.

BLS (Bureau of Labor Statistics). 2009-10. Counselors. In *Occupational outlook handbook, 2009-10 ed.* http://www.bls.gov/oco/ocos067.htm. (Accessed January 8, 2010).

Bobby CL. 2009. *Accreditation of counselor education programs: CACREP.* Presentation made to the IOM Committee on Qualification of Professionals Providing Mental Health Services Under TRICARE, April 9.

Bradley RW, Cox JA. 2001. Counseling: Evolution of the profession. In *The handbook of counseling,* edited by Locke DC, Myers JE, Herr EL. Thousand Oaks, CA: Sage. Pp. 27-41.

CACREP (Council for Accreditation of Counseling and Related Educational Programs). 2008. *CACREP 2001 standards.* http://www.cacrep.org/2001Standards.html. (Accessed June 22, 2009).

CACREP. 2009a. *2009 standards.* http://www.cacrep.org/2009standards.html. (Accessed August 6, 2009).

CACREP. 2009b. *CACREP accreditation manual. 2009 standards.* Alexandria, VA: Council for Accreditation of Counseling and Related Educational Programs.

CACREP. 2009c. *Directory of accredited programs.* http://www.cacrep.org/directory.html. (Accessed August 6, 2009).

CCNE (Commission on Collegiate Nursing Education). 2009. *CCNE accreditation.* http://www.aacn.nche.edu/accreditation/. (Accessed November 5, 2009).

CHEA (Council on Higher Education Accreditation). 2009. *Accreditation, students and society: talking points.* http://www.chea.org/pdf/2009_Talking_Points.pdf. (Accessed November 7, 2009).

Chronister J, Chou CC, Chan J. 2009. The roles and functions of professional counselors. In *The professional counselor's desk reference*, edited by Marini I, Stebnicki M. New York: Springer Publishing Co. Pp. 15-25.

Clawson TW. 2009. *Qualifications of professionals providing mental health counseling services under TRICARE.* Presentation to the IOM Committee on Qualification of Professionals Providing Mental Health Services Under TRICARE, April 9.

CORE (Council on Rehabilitation Education). 2008a. *CORE self-study document: Rehabilitation counselor education accreditation evaluation,* rev. 04/08. http://www.core-rehab.org/NonManDocs/coreSSD.608.DOC. (Accessed January 10, 2010).

CORE. 2008b. *CORE standards compliance checklist.* http://www.core-rehab.org/NonManDocs/c-coorappenB.608.doc. (Accessed January 10, 2010).

Corey G, Corey MS, Callanan P. 2006. *Issues and ethics in the helping professions,* 7th ed. Belmont, CA: Brooks/Cole (Thomson).

CRCC (Commission on Rehabilitation Counselor Certification). 2009a. *CRC Certification Guide.* http://www.crccertification.com/filebin/pdf/CRC_Certification_Guide200908.pdf. (Accessed October 16, 2009).

CRCC. 2009b. *Welcome to the CRCC.* http://www.crccertification.com/. (Accessed October 16, 2009).

CSWE (Council on Social Work Education). 2008. *Educational policy and accreditation standards.* http://www.cswe.org/File.aspx?id=13780. (Accessed June 22, 2009).

Department of Veterans Affairs, Veterans Health Administration. 2008. Credentialing and privileging. In *VHA Handbook* 1100.19, November 14. http://www1.va.gov/vhapublications/ViewPublication.asp?pub_ID=1806. (Accessed September 8, 2009).

DOD (Department of Defense). 2004. *Military Health System (MHS) clinical quality assurance (CQA) program regulation.* DOD 6025-13r, June 1. http://www.dtic.mil/whs/directives/corres/pdf/602513r.pdf. (Accessed September 8, 2009).

DOD. 2006. *Aspects of the use of licensed professional counselors in the Military Health System. Report to Congress.* Transmittal letter, August 28. http://www.tricare.mil/planning/congress/downloads/2006/new/Licensed-Mental.pdf. (Accessed October 20, 2009).

DOD Directive Number 6025.13. 1995. *Clinical quality management program (CQMP) in the military health services system (MHSS),* July 20. http://www.tricare.mil/ops/P3C1AA.PDF. (Accessed November 7, 2009).

Duncan BL, Miller SD, Sparks JA. 2004. *The heroic client: A revolutionary way to improve effectiveness through client directed, outcome-informed therapy.* New York: John Wiley & Son.

Gibson RL, Mitchell MH. 2008. *Introduction to counseling and guidance,* 7th ed. Upper Saddle River, NJ: Merrill/Prentice-Hall.

Gladding ST. 2009. *Counseling: A comprehensive profession*, 6th ed. Englewood Cliffs, NJ: Merrill/Prentice-Hall.

Gross SJ. 1979. The myth of professional licensing. *American Psychologist* 33(11): 1009-1016.

Hershenson DB, Berger GP. 2001. The state of community counseling: A survey of directors of CACREP-accredited programs. *Journal of Counseling & Development* 79(2):188-193.

HHS (Department of Health and Human Services). 1996. *Review of the policies and procedures for medical personnel credentialing and privileging at the Indian Health Service.* National Institutes of Health, and Health Resources and Services Administration, December 16. http://oig.hhs.gov/oas/reports/phs/c9400006.htm. (Accessed April 22, 2010).

Hoge MA, Jacobs S, Belitsky R, Migdole S. 2002. Graduate education and training for contemporary behavioral health practice. *Administration and Policy in Mental Health* 29(4/5):335-357.

Hosie T. 1995. Counseling specialties: A case of basic preparation rather than advanced specialization. *Journal of Counseling & Development* 74(2):177-180.

IOM (Institute of Medicine). 2006. *Improving the quality of health care for mental and substance-use conditions: Quality chasm series.* Washington, DC: The National Academies Press.

LCME (Liaison Committee on Medical Education). 2008. *LCME accreditation standards.* http://www.lcme.org/functionsnarrative.htm#educational%20program. (Accessed June 22, 2009).

Manderscheid RW, Berry JT (Eds.). 2004. *Mental health, United States, 2004.* Rockville, MD: Department of Health and Human Services.

Myers J. 1995. Specialties in counseling: Rich heritage or force for fragmentation? *Journal of Counseling & Development* 74(2):115-116.

NBCC (National Board for Certified Counselors). 2009a. *About us.* http://www.nbcc.org/whoWeAre/About.aspx. (Accessed October 20, 2009).

NBCC. 2009b. *Certified Clinical Mental Health Counselor credential for counselors who hold the NCC credential: 2010 Application.* http://www.nbcc.org/AssetManagerFiles/apps/ccmhce-app_T10.pdf. (Accessed October 21, 2009).

NBCC. 2009c. *Clinical mental health counselors modified* activities detailed content outline.* Information provided in response to a request from the Committee on the Qualifications of Professionals Providing Mental Health Counseling Services Under TRICARE. Dated August 13.

NBCC. 2009d. *National Clinical Mental Health Counseling Examination (NCMHCE) development process.* Information provided in response to a request from the Committee on the Qualifications of Professionals Providing Mental Health Counseling Services Under TRICARE. Dated August 13.

NBCC. 2010. *The National Certified Counselor (NCC) credential and the National Counselor Examination (NCE).* http://www.nbcc.org/certifications/ncc/Default.aspx. (Accessed January 10, 2010).

NCQA (National Committee for Quality Assurance). 2009. *HEDIS & quality measurement.* http://www.ncqa.org/tabid/59/Default.aspx. (Accessed October 16, 2009).

Neukrug E. 2003. *The work of the counselor: An introduction to the counseling profession,* 2nd ed. Pacific Grove, CA: Brooks/Cole.

Neukrug E, Milliken T, Walden S. 2001. Ethics complaints against credentialed counselors: An updated survey of state licensing boards. *Counselor Education and Supervision* 41:57-70.

Reaves RP. 2003. *Avoiding liability in mental health practice.* Montgomery, AL: Association of State and Provincial Psychology Boards.

Remley TP, Herlihy B. 2010. *Ethical, legal, and professional issues in counseling,* 3rd ed. Upper Saddle River, NJ: Pearson.

Sales A. 2007. *Rehabilitation counseling: An empowerment perspective.* Austin, TX: Pro-Ed.

Schweiger WK, Henderson DA, Clawson TW. 2008. *Counselor preparation: Programs, faculty, trends,* 12th ed. New York: Routledge.

Shaffer I. 2009. *Master's-prepared clinicians delivering mental health care.* 2009. Presentation to the Committee on the Qualifications of Professionals Providing Mental Health Counseling Services Under TRICARE, July 7.

State of Delaware. 2010. *Department of State: Division of Professional Regulation: Mental health and chemical dependency professionals, FAQ.* http://dpr.delaware.gov/boards/profcounselors/faqs.shtml. (Accessed January 7, 2010).

Sweeney T. 1995. Accreditation, credentialing, professionalization: The role of specialties. *Journal of Counseling & Development* 74(2):117-125.

Sweeney T. 2001. Counseling: Historical origins and philosophical roots. *The handbook of counseling,* edited by Locke D, Myers J, Herr E. Thousand Oaks, CA: Sage. Pp. 3-26.

URAC. 2009. *General questions about URAC accreditation.* http://www.urac.org/accreditation/. (Accessed October 16, 2009).

Van Horne BA. 2004. Psychology licensing board disciplinary actions: The realities. *Professional Psychology: Research and Practice* 35(2):170-178.

# 4

# Independent and Supervised Practice of Counselors in Other Health-Care Systems

As part of the committee's statement of task, the Department of Defense requested that it assess the extent to which mental health counselors are authorized to practice independently under some federal programs other than TRICARE and under the Federal Employee Health Benefits Program (FEHBP). It was also asked to identify the states that had laws requiring private insurers to cover, or offer coverage of, the services of licensed mental health counselors. This chapter addresses those topics.

## INDEPENDENT AND SUPERVISED PRACTICE UNDER OTHER FEDERAL PROGRAMS

The statement of task identified four federal programs for attention: Medicare, the Department of Veterans Affairs (VA) program, the Indian Health Service (IHS) program, and Head Start (HS). The text below briefly reviews their policies and those of the US Public Health Service (PHS) regarding the practice of counselors.

### Medicare

#### *Practice Under Medicare*

Medicare is a federally administered health insurance program for people 65 years old or older, people under 65 years old who have specified disabilities, and people of any age who have permanent kidney failure (CMS, 2009). The program covers the cost of mental health–care visits with physicians, clinical psychologists, clinical social workers, clinical nurse specialists, nurse practitioners, and physician's assistants (CMS, 2002). Those health-care professionals are recognized as independent providers of mental health services under Medicare regulations.

Medicare does not recognize licensed professional counselors as independent providers, so they are not directly reimbursed through the program. Provisions in several bills that have been introduced in the House of Representatives and the Senate would have added counselors and some other mental health professionals to those eligible to provide services (CRS, 2007), but the provisions have not been enacted into law. As of October 1, 2009, bills that would grant that authority were under consideration in both chambers (HR 1693 and S 671).

Medicare beneficiaries can receive services from counselors in two ways. They can visit practitioners and pay for the expense out of pocket, or the counselors can provide treatment through the Part B "incident to" clause. The latter method allows counselors to bill Medicare through physicians or psychologists. To be covered by the clause, a service must be an integral, although incidental, part of a physician's or psychologist's services; the counselor must work in the same facility as a physician or psychologist (as either an employee or independent contractor of the physician or psychologist or the facility); and the counselor must be under the supervision of the physician or psychologist. Supervision means that "the physician/psychologist must be present in the facility and immediately available to provide assistance and direction while the aide is performing services" (ACA, 2009a). The physician, psychologist, or facility bills Medicare for the service, and the counselor is paid as an employee or contractor of the physician, psychologist, or facility.

### *Association Between Independent Practice Authority Under the Medicare Program and Under TRICARE*

The committee's statement of task directed it to review the relationship, if any, between recognition of mental health professions under the Medicare program and independent practice authority for such professions under the TRICARE program. Only one non-doctoral-level mental health profession—clinical social work—has been granted independent practice authority by both TRICARE and Medicare. Clinical social workers were first granted authority under TRICARE in the FY 1983 Department of Defense Authorization Act (Public Law 97-252) and were later granted recognition under Medicare in the Omnibus Budget Reconciliation Act of 1989 (Public Law 101-239). Congress directed the authority to be granted in both circumstances. Marriage and family therapists have been granted independent practice authority only under TRICARE, through a provision of the FY 1991 Department of Defense Authorization Act (Public Law 101-510); they have not been granted recognition under Medicare. Licensed professional counselors have not been granted independent practice authority under either TRICARE or Medicare.

### Department of Veterans Affairs

VA, through programs of the Veterans Health Administration, provides a comprehensive array of health-care services to about 7.9 million enrollees (VA, 2009). In December 2006, the Veterans Benefits, Healthcare, and Information Technology Act was signed into law (Public Law 109-461). It established the recognition of mental health counselors as mental health–care specialists under health-care programs operated by VA. It also established the recognition of licensed marriage and family therapists as mental health–care providers. Although VA has long employed rehabilitation counselors to provide readjustment-counseling services to veterans, it did not previously recognize these professional groups. The new law allows VA to hire licensed mental health counselors at the same level as clinical social workers and allows counselors to apply for supervisory positions that are open to clinical social workers and marriage and family therapists. Rather than placing them in the same occupational category as other mental health professionals, the VA Under Secretary for Health approved, in February 2009, the creation of a new occupational category or categories for licensed professional counselors and marriage and family therapists to be hired by VA (ACA, 2009b). Details of those categories had not been established at the time the present report was completed.

### Indian Health Service

IHS is an agency in the Department of Health and Human Services (HHS). It is the principal federal health-care provider and health advocate for American Indians and Alaska Natives and is responsible for providing federal health services to about 1.9 million people who belong to 562 federally recognized tribes in 35 states. The goal of IHS is "to assure that comprehensive, culturally acceptable personal and public health services are available and accessible to American Indian and Alaska Native people" (IHS, 2009c). Because this population experiences considerable disparities with regard to psychological health compared with the general population and because over one-third of the service demands in IHS facilities are related to mental health and substance abuse, IHS behavioral health programs are particularly important to the population.

IHS will accept a state license and the stipulated scope of practice for the license as criteria for the delivery of services in IHS facilities. In addition, individual credentialing agencies can further define and limit the scope of practice for some professionals, including advanced-practice nurses and other allied-health professionals in the federal system. Over 60% of mental health treatment and almost all substance-abuse counseling takes place at the tribal level (IHS, 2009a). IHS credentialing standards serve as the base guidelines for tribes, but they are able to establish additional or different standards if they choose. Regardless of the standards used, the focus is always on the scope of practice, particularly at the credentialing level.

Behavioral health programs in IHS include community-oriented clinical and preventive services. The delivery of needed services is complex, however, and often divided among tribal, federal, state, local, and community-based providers. In addition, the availability of services varies among communities; those who live in rural areas are most adversely affected by problems of availability and lack of appropriate care. Overall, the behavioral health needs of this population are largely unmet, and adequate services are scarce and access to appropriate care difficult and expensive (IHS, 2009a).

The policy of IHS is to use interdisciplinary mental health teams that comprise representatives of several mental health disciplines to provide comprehensive services to the American Indian and Alaska Native population. Mental health providers identified in IHS include psychiatrists, psychologists, psychiatric nurses, psychiatric social workers, other social scientists, and mental health technicians. IHS policies stipulate that all mental health staff working in IHS facilities must meet the minimum educational requirements set forth by the Civil Service or

Commissioned Corps. Mental health professionals and consultants must also be licensed in accordance with existing PHS requirements, which stipulate that all health-care providers must be licensed, certified, or registered in their disciplines (PHS-CC, 2008a). Clinical privileges are recommended for mental health technicians, mental health counselors, and psychiatric nurses and allow them to provide clinical mental health services independently of physician supervision.

Licensing and credentialing standards for mental health professionals in IHS center on educational requirements, but clinical privileging standards have also been established for IHS providers on the basis of licensure, training, experience, and current competence "for all individuals who are permitted by law and by a facility to provide patient care services independently in a facility whether or not they are members of the medical staff" (IHS, 2009b).

Clinical privileges are granted and maintained on the basis of demonstrated clinical competence, including an assessment of relevant findings from quality-assurance activities, peer recommendations, measured assurance that people consistently provide services within the scope of their privileges, a review of privileges at least every 2 years, and established procedures for the denial, limitation, or change in clinical privileges granted to any health-care provider. In addition to retaining their clinical privileges, mental health professionals must participate in continuing education to maintain their licensure and to continue providing services in IHS facilities.

## Head Start

HS is a national program administered by HHS that "promotes school readiness by enhancing the social and cognitive development of children through the provision of educational, health, nutritional, social and other services to enrolled children and families" (HHS, 2009). Although the program does not have a formal policy regarding the use and independent practice of licensed professional counselors, it follows the rules of the states in which mental health services are being provided. HS provides grants to local agencies that agree to follow HS regulations in implementing their programs. The grantees determine how they will use their grant funds on the basis of local needs and resources but must ensure that they meet HS regulations regarding making mental health consultation available onsite. HS program-performance standards (federal regulations) require that a grantee's mental health services be supported by staff or consultants who are licensed or certified mental health professionals with experience and expertise in serving young children and their families.

Programs must recognize that state licensure and certification systems review a professional's training and experience and describe the scope of services that a professional is qualified to provide to children and families in the states. HS grantees are not required to provide all mental health services that a child may need but are encouraged to identify local mental health resources that can provide such services. Overall, HS does not act as a primary provider of mental health services but rather as a funder of entities that may then contract themselves out to provide services. Some other entities that may fund provision of services under specific circumstances—Medicaid, for example—may have their own policies and procedures that drive the scope of practice or billing rules.

## US Public Health Service

The Commissioned Corps of PHS is one of the seven uniformed services of the United States. Among its primary missions is to provide health care to underserved populations. Its officers are placed in various career fields—such as medicine, nursing, dentistry, and environmental health—depending on their training (PHS-CC, 2009a). One field, health services, includes a variety of professionals, including such clinical specialists as psychologists, social workers, physician assistants, and optometrists and such nonclinical specialists as hospital administrators (PHS-CC, 2008c).

The Corps has a goal of expanding its active-duty strength to 6,600 officers. Some 5% of that number, or 330, are to be officers in the mental health functional group (PHS-CC, 2009b). As of May 15, 2007, the Corps had 108 clinical social workers and 14 clinical psychologists in its health-services field (PHS-CC, 2007). Psychiatrists and psychiatric nurses also serve in the Corps, but their numbers are not publicly available (PHS-CC, 2009c). The title "licensed professional counselor" is not listed among its professional categories.

## INDEPENDENT AND SUPERVISED PRACTICE UNDER THE FEDERAL EMPLOYEE HEALTH BENEFITS PROGRAM

### Overview of the Program

The FEHBP was established by law in 1959 and became active in 1960 (OPM, 2009d).[1] It is administered by the Office of Personnel Management (OPM) and provides federal employees and eligible family members with a variety of privately run, government-subsidized insurance plans. Among the plan types are fee-for-service (FFS) plans, high-deductible health plans, and health maintenance organization (HMO) plans (OPM, 2009c). The selection of plans available to a particular employee depends both on geographic area and on the employing government organization.

Plans may not turn down employees or eligible family members because of preexisting medical conditions (OPM, 2009f). In general, costs of the plan are split between the employee and the federal government; the government pays the smaller of 75% of the chosen plan cost or 72% of the average plan cost of all FEHBP enrollees (OPM, 2009b). Most federal employees are eligible for the FEHBP; exceptions are made for intermittent or temporary employees and employees of specific organizations, such as the Tennessee Valley Authority (OPM, 2009a). On retirement, qualified employees may continue enrollment in their current plan (OPM, 2009f).

The FEHBP offers 10 FFS benefit plans that are available nationwide to all enrollees: the American Postal Workers Union "high," Blue Cross and Blue Shield "standard" and "basic," Government Employees Hospital Association "standard" and "high," Mail Handlers "standard" and "value," National Association of Letter Carriers "high," and Special Agents Mutual Benefit Association "standard" and "high." Each of those plans provides comprehensive coverage and has separate provider networks for which in-network providers have reduced costs. All plans offer international coverage (OPM, 2009f).

Four other FFS benefit plans available nationwide through the FEHBP are sponsored by employee organizations, and enrollment is strictly limited to members of the organizations: Association "high,"

---

[1]The FEHBP was established by Public Law 86-382. Current laws and regulations are found in 5 USC Chapter 89, 5 CFR Part 890, and 48 CFR Chapter 16.

Foreign Service "high," Panama Canal Area "high," and Rural Carrier "high" (OPM, 2009f).

Finally, the FEHBP includes a set of plans that are available only to subscribers in particular states. The number of plans and the services offered vary widely among the states. For example, eligible California residents have a choice of plans available through Aetna, Blue Cross, Blue Shield, Health Net, Kaiser Foundation, PacifiCare, and UnitedHealthcare; Texas residents have access to Aetna, Firstcare, Humana, PacifiCare, and UnitedHealthcare plans; and Pennsylvania residents can choose from Aetna, Geisinger, HealthAmerica, Keystone, and University of Pittsburgh Medical Center plans (OPM, 2009g). The coverage area, including the number of states where coverage is offered, varies among plans. Altius Health Plans, for example, limits coverage to subscribers in particular sections of Utah, Idaho, and Wyoming, while Aetna Healthfund provides insurance plans in all 50 states and the District of Columbia (Table 4.1).

The mental health services and providers covered by the plans differ by care organization, options purchased, and the state in which the plan was purchased. It may also vary from year to year.

## Program Policies Regarding Independent Practice

The law governing the FEHBP lists licensed health-care providers whom plan enrollees must be free to see without physician referral or supervision (Table 4.2; 5 USC § 8902(k)(1)). HMO plans are exempted from the rule because a key feature of them is that a primary-care provider coordinates and refers specialist care (5 USC § 8902(k)(3)). Qualified clinical social workers—defined as those who have met state licensing requirements, national certification requirements in the absence of state licensing procedures, or "equivalent requirements" as determined by OPM—are among the providers whose services without physician supervision or referral must be covered (5 USC § 8901(11)). Except in states designated by OPM as underserved (Table 4.3), FEHBP plans are not explicitly required to cover licensed professional counselors, although the law allows insurance plans to voluntarily cover other health professionals' (including counselors') services without physician supervision or referral, provided that the professionals are appropriately licensed or certified by state or federal law (5 USC § 8902(k)(1) and (2)). In underserved states, FFS, but not HMO, plans must cover all state-

**TABLE 4.1** Coverage of Licensed Mental Health Counselors in FEHBP Nationwide and Selected State Insurance Plans

| 2010 Federal Insurance Plans | FEHBP Plan Codes | Licensed Mental Health Counselors Coverage | Plan Details (Provider Definitions or Listed Benefits) |
|---|---|---|---|
| NATIONWIDE FEE-FOR-SERVICE PLANS—OPEN TO ALL | | | |
| Blue Cross and Blue Shield Service Benefit Plan | 10, 11 | Yes | Mental health or substance-abuse professional: a professional who is licensed by the state where the care is provided to provide mental health or substance-abuse services within the scope of the license<br><br>Benefits include professional services, including individual or group therapy, provided by *licensed professional mental health practitioners* and substance-abuse practitioners when acting within the scope of their licenses |
| Government Employees Hospital Association Benefit and High Deductible Health Plans | 31, 34 | Yes[a] | Benefits include individual or group therapy by psychiatrists, psychologists, clinical social workers, *licensed professional counselors*, and marriage and family therapists |
| National Association of Letter Carriers | 32 | No[a] | Benefits include outpatient professional services, including individual or group therapy by such providers as psychiatrists, psychologists, and clinical social workers |
| Mail Handlers Benefit Plan Value and Consumer Option | 41, 45, 48 | Yes | Benefits include outpatient professional services, including individual or group therapy by providers approved by the managed in-network vendor; may include services by a *licensed professional counselor* or licensed marriage and family therapist |

*continued*

**TABLE 4.1** Continued

| 2010 Federal Insurance Plans | FEHBP Plan Codes | Licensed Mental Health Counselors Coverage | Plan Details (Provider Definitions or Listed Benefits) |
|---|---|---|---|
| Special Agents Mutual Benefit Association | 44 | Yes[a] | Benefits include outpatient professional services by such providers as psychiatrists, psychologists, and clinical social workers |
| American Postal Workers Union Health Plan | 47 | Yes | Benefits include professional services, including individual or group therapy by such providers as psychiatrists, psychologists, licensed social workers, and licensed intensive outpatient treatment centers |
| NATIONWIDE FEE-FOR-SERVICE PLANS—OPEN ONLY TO SPECIFIC GROUPS | | | |
| Rural Carrier Benefit Plan Specific Areas | 38 | Yes[a] | Qualified clinical psychologist: a person who has earned a doctoral or master's clinical degree in psychology or an allied discipline and who is licensed or certified in the state where services are performed; this presumes that a licensed person has demonstrated to the satisfaction of state licensing officials that he or she, by virtue of academic and clinical experience, is qualified to provide psychological services in the state |
| Foreign Service Benefit Plan Specific Areas | 40 | Yes | Qualified clinical psychologist: a person who has earned a doctoral or master's clinical degree in psychology or an allied discipline and who is licensed or certified in the state where services are performed (such as licensed professional counselors) |

**TABLE 4.1** Continued

| 2010 Federal Insurance Plans | FEHBP Plan Codes | Licensed Mental Health Counselors Coverage | Plan Details (Provider Definitions or Listed Benefits) |
|---|---|---|---|
| Association Benefit Plan Specific Areas | 42 | Yes | Qualified clinical psychologist: a person who has earned a doctoral or master's clinical degree in psychology or an allied discipline and who is licensed or certified in the state where services are performed; this presumes that a licensed person has demonstrated to the satisfaction of state licensing officials that he or she, by virtue of academic and clinical experience, is qualified to provide psychological services in the state |
| Panama Canal Area Benefit Plan Specific Areas | 43 | No[a] | Benefits include outpatient services, including individual or group therapy by such providers as psychiatrists, psychologists, and clinical social workers |
| SELECTED STATE-SPECIFIC INURANCE PLANS | | | |
| UnitedHealthcare Insurance Company, Inc., serving AR, AZ, CA, CO, DC, FL, GA, IA, IL, KS, LA, MD, MO, MS, NC, NM, NV, OH, OK, OR, RI, TN, TX, VA, WA, WI | E9 | Yes[a] | Benefits include professional services, including individual or group therapy by such providers as psychiatrists, psychologists, and clinical social workers |

*continued*

**TABLE 4.1** Continued

| 2010 Federal Insurance Plans | FEHBP Plan Codes | Licensed Mental Health Counselors Coverage | Plan Details (Provider Definitions or Listed Benefits) |
|---|---|---|---|
| Aetna HealthFund, serving AK, AL, AR, AZ, CA, CO, CT, DC, DE, FL, GA, HI, IA, ID, IL, IN, KS, KY, LA, MA, MD, ME, MI, MN, MO, MS, MT, NC, ND, NE, NH, NJ, NM, NV, NY, OH, OK, OR, PA, RI, SC, SD, TN, TX, UT, VA, VT, WA, WI, WV, WY | 22 | Yes[a] | Benefits include individual and group therapy performed by such licensed providers as psychiatrists, psychologists, and clinical social workers |
| Altius Health Plans, serving Utah (northern and southern parts of Utah), Idaho (Boise and eastern parts of Idaho), and Wyoming (Uinta County) | 9K | Yes[a] | Benefits include professional services, including individual or group therapy by such providers as psychiatrists, psychologists, and clinical social workers |

[a]Publicly available sources did not specify whether the services of licensed mental health counselors were covered. Listed information was obtained via telephone calls to company representatives.

**TABLE 4.2** Licensed Health-Care Providers Whose Services Must Be Covered by FEHBP Plans Without Requiring Physician Referral or Supervision[a]

| | |
|---|---|
| Clinical psychologist | Nursing-school–administered clinic |
| Optometrist | Nurse practitioner or clinical specialist |
| Nurse midwife | Qualified clinical social worker |

[a]This list is found under 5 USC § 8902(k)(1). HMOs are exempt from these requirements, under 5 USC § 8902(k)(3).

**TABLE 4.3** States Designated as Medically Underserved by OPM for 2009[a]

| | | |
|---|---|---|
| Alabama | Louisiana | North Dakota |
| Arizona | Mississippi | South Carolina |
| Idaho | Missouri | South Dakota |
| Illinois | Montana | Wyoming |
| Kentucky | New Mexico | |

[a]Determinations of underserved status are made annually by OPM. The definition of *medically underserved* is found in 6 USC § 254e.

licensed medical providers although the law does not indicate whether physician supervision or referral is necessary (OPM, 2009e).

Because there is no federal licensing process for mental health counselors, an FEHBP plan that wishes to recognize counselors can do so only in accordance with the laws and regulations of the states where they practice. The Foreign Service Benefit Plan, for example, is an FFS FEHBP plan that includes state-licensed professional counselors among its covered providers (AFSPA, 2009, p. 10). Being an FFS plan, it allows enrollees to visit any covered provider, including counselors, without first obtaining a referral from a physician. That particular plan, however, requires preauthorization for any mental health treatment besides medication management (AFSPA, 2009, p. 48). Table 4.1 lists the federal FFS plans and a sample of state plans and shows which plans include coverage for licensed mental health counselors.

### State Laws, Regulations, and Policies Regarding Independent Practice

States differ in their laws, regulations, and policies regarding the independent practice of counselors. An April 2009 presentation to the committee noted that 14 states require health plans to cover the services of licensed counselors and another six require plans to offer coverage; these are listed in Table 4.4 (Kaplan, 2009). Arkansas and Michigan laws include so-called "any-willing-provider"[2] provisions that include counselors.

More generally, the scope of practice and range of services allowed vary in both their details and specificity. Alabama law, for example, provides relatively general guidance, stipulating that

> [t]he use of specific methods, techniques, or modalities within the practice of a Licensed Professional Counselor is restricted to counselors appropriately trained in the use of these methods, techniques, or modalities. A licensed professional counselor or associate licensed counselor shall not attempt to diagnose, prescribe for, treat, or advise a client with reference to problems or complaints falling outside the boundaries of counseling services. (Alabama Board of Examiners in Counseling, 2003)

Nebraska, in contrast, allows only persons who hold the more rigorous Independent Mental Health Practitioner license to perform diagnoses. That license requires 3,000 hours of experience under supervision, "one-half of which is comprised of experience with clients diagnosed under the major mental illness or disorder category" (Nebraska Department of Health and Human Services, 2007). The illnesses and disorders are defined elsewhere as schizophrenia, major depressive disorder, bipolar disorder, delusional disorder, psychotic disorder, panic disorder, and obsessive-compulsive disorder (Nebraska Department of Health and Human Services Regulation and Licensure, 2004).

The array of services offered is constrained in some states. For example, California, which is scheduled to begin to license counselors in 2011, does not include the assessment or treatment of couples or families in a professional clinical counselor's scope of practice unless the counselor "has completed all of the following additional training and education, beyond the minimum training and education required for licensure" (California State Senate, Senate Bill 788, 2009).

---

[2]Any-willing-provider legislation requires that health plans accept any health-care provider who agrees to conform to the plans' conditions, terms, and reimbursement rates (Carroll and Ambrose, 2002).

**TABLE 4.4** States That Require Coverage or the Offering of Coverage of Counselors' Services

| | | |
|---|---|---|
| States That Require Coverage | | |
| Arkansas | New Hampshire | Virginia |
| Connecticut | Rhode Island | Washington |
| Maryland | South Dakota | Wyoming |
| Massachusetts | Texas | |
| Montana | Utah | |
| States That Require That Coverage Be Offered | | |
| Illinois | Louisiana | Missouri |
| Kansas | Maine | Vermont |
| States with Any-Willing-Provider Laws Addressing Counselors | | |
| Arkansas | Michigan | |

SOURCE: Adapted from Kaplan (2009).

Terminology also varies. Notably, Maine licenses Professional Counselors and Clinical Professional Counselors: both are permitted to "engage in private/independent practice" (Maine Office of Licensing and Registration, 2009), but only persons holding clinical licenses may "diagnose and treat mental health disorders" (Maine Revised Statues, Title 32, Chapter 119, § 13858).

All states allow counselors to practice independently at some level of licensure. Supervised practice is required for persons who hold "conditional," "intern," "provisional," and like-titled licenses in the states that offer them. Those licenses are intended for persons who are beginning their professional careers and seeking to accumulate the experience needed for higher-level licenses and national certifications. Rules regarding whether counselors can perform diagnoses are more complicated. Most states explicitly include diagnosis in the scope of practice delineated in law or regulation. Three—Georgia, Idaho, and Illinois—do not use the term, and this leads to uncertainty. Maine and New Mexico permit those holding clinical licenses to perform diagnoses, Indiana prohibits counselors from making diagnoses but allows them to perform classifications according to the *Diagnostic and Statistical Manual of Mental Disorders,* and Nebraska permits only those holding licensure as a Licensed Independent Mental Health Practitioner to perform diagnoses.

## REFERENCES

ACA (American Counseling Association). 2009a. *Frequently asked questions: Medicare. (2.19.09)*. http://www.counseling.org/Files/FD.ashx?guid=1b2019e5-1ed1-4c9f-b0bb-9b92298fa368. (Accessed October 12, 2009).

ACA. 2009b. *Progress on implementation of new Veterans Affairs law*. http://www.counseling.org/PublicPolicy/PositionPapers.aspx?AGuid=682a95b9-d0be-4f6d-982a-97fa7ed80737. (Accessed October 28, 2009).

AFSPA (American Foreign Service Protective Association). 2009. Foreign service benefit plans. In *Center for Retirement and Insurance Services*. Washington, DC: US Office of Personnel Management. http://www.opm.gov/insure/health/planinfo/2009/brochures/72-001.pdf. (Accessed October 28, 2009).

Alabama Board of Examiners in Counseling. 2003. Definitions and clarification of terms. In *Administrative Rules*, Chapter 255-X-2. http://www.abec.state.al.us/PDFs/255_X_2_JULY_03.pdf. (Accessed January 8, 2010).

Carroll A, Ambrose JM. 2002. Any-willing-provider laws: Their financial effects on HMOs. *Journal of Health Politics, Policy and Law* 27(6):927-945.

CMS (Centers for Medicare and Medicaid Services). 2002. *Medicare and your mental health benefits*. Bethesda, MD: National Institute of Mental Health.

CMS. 2009. *What is Medicare?* http://www.medicare.gov/Publications/Pubs/pdf/11306.pdf. (Accessed October 12, 2009).

CRS (Congressional Research Service). 2007. *The Mental Health Parity Act. A Legislative History*. CRS Report for Congress. Order Code RL33820. Washington, DC: US Government Printing Office.

HHS (Department of Health and Human Services). 2009. *About the Office of Head Start*. http://www.acf.hhs.gov/programs/ohs/about/. (Accessed October 12, 2009).

IHS (Indian Health Service). 2009a. *Behavioral health*. http://info.ihs.gov/Bhealth.asp. (Accessed October 28, 2009).

IHS. 2009b. Mental health program. In *Indian health manual*. Rockville, MD: Department of Health and Human Services. Part 3, Chapter 14.

IHS. 2009c. *Indian Health Service introduction*. http://www.ihs.gov/PublicInfo/PublicAffairs/Welcome_Info/IHSintro.asp. (Accessed October 28, 2009).

Kaplan D. 2009. *Licensed mental health counselors and the TRICARE Program*. Presentation to the Institute of Medicine Committee on the Committee on the Qualifications of Professionals Providing Mental Health Counseling Services Under TRICARE, April 9. http://www.iom.edu/~/media/Files/Activity%20Files/MentalHealth/TRICAREMentalHealth/KaplanIOMpresentation.ashx. (Accessed November 7, 2009).

Maine Office of Licensing and Registration. 2009. *Board of Counseling Professionals Licensure—Frequently Asked Questions*. http://www.maine.gov/pfr/professionallicensing/professions/counselors/faq_licensee.htm. (Accessed October 12, 2009).

Nebraska Department of Health and Human Services. 2007. *Mental health practice*. http://www.hhs.state.ne.us/crl/mhcs/mental/mentalhealth.htm. (Accessed October 12, 2009).

Nebraska Department of Health and Human Services Regulation and Licensure. 2004. *Licensure of mental health practitioners and the certification of marriage and family therapists, professional counselors and social workers.* Title 172, Chapter 94, July 28. http://www.sos.state.ne.us/rules-and-regs/regsearch/Rules/Health_and_Human_Services_System/Title-172/Chapter-94.pdf. (Accessed October 12, 2009).

OPM (Office of Personnel Management). 2009a. *Federal Employees Health Benefits Program handbook: Eligibility for Health Benefits.* http://www.opm.gov/insure/health/reference/handbook/fehb06.asp. (Accessed October 28, 2009).

OPM. 2009b. *Federal Employees Health Benefits Program Handbook: Government's Share.* http://www.opm.gov/insure/health/reference/handbook/fehb03.asp#govshare. (Accessed October 28, 2009).

OPM. 2009c. *Federal Employees Health Benefits Program Handbook: Health Plans.* http://www.opm.gov/insure/health/reference/handbook/fehb05.asp#top. (Accessed October 28, 2009).

OPM. 2009d. *Federal Employees Health Benefits Program Handbook: Laws and Regulations.* http://www.opm.gov/insure/health/reference/handbook/fehb01.asp#lawandregs. (Accessed October 28, 2009).

OPM. 2009e. *Federal Employees Health Benefits Program Handbook: Payment of Benefits in Medically Underserved Areas.* http://www.opm.gov/insure/health/reference/handbook/fehb05.asp#paymentunder. (Accessed October 28, 2009).

OPM. 2009f. *2009 Guide to federal benefits for federal civilian employees.* http://sig.nfc.usda.gov/dprs/RI%2070-01%202009.pdf. (Accessed October 28, 2009).

OPM. 2009g. *Federal Employees Health Benefits Program: Choose a Plan & Enroll.* http://www.opm.gov/insure/health/planinfo/index.asp. (Accessed October 28, 2009).

PHS-CC (US Public Health Service Commissioned Corps). 2007. *CPO Forum: USPHS Scientific and Training Symposium.* Presentation by the Chief Health Services Officer. http://usphs-hso.org/cpo/CPO_COA2007.pdf. (Accessed October 28, 2009).

PHS-CC. 2008a. *Mental health/behavioral health requirements.* http://www.usphs.gov/profession/behavioral/requirements.aspx. (Accessed October 28, 2009).

PHS-CC. 2008b. *Profession: Health service.* http://www.usphs.gov/profession/healthservices/activities.aspx. (Accessed October 28, 2009).

PHS-CC. 2009a. *Profession.* http://www.usphs.gov/Profession/. (Accessed October 28, 2009).

PHS-CC. 2009b. *Career and assignment manager (CAM) Teams—FAQs.* http://www.usphs.gov/transformation/CAM.aspx. (Accessed October 28, 2009).

PHS-CC. 2009c. *USPHS physicians professional advisory committee.* Minutes from January 28 meeting. http://usphs-ppac.org/PPAC_Meeting_%20Minutes_1-28-09_DRAFT.pdf. (Accessed October 28, 2009).

# 5

# Research Regarding the Determinants of High-Quality Mental Health Care

In this chapter, the committee reviews existing standards and expectations for the delivery of high-quality mental health care with special reference to psychosocial services relevant to the most prevalent conditions in the TRICARE beneficiary population. The statement of task that guided the committee's work requested that it review the scientific literature regarding the quality and effectiveness of care provided by licensed mental health counselors. The committee was also asked to offer recommendations regarding modifications of current TRICARE policy with respect to allowing licensed mental health counselors to practice independently. Because the policy is built around TRICARE's system of quality management through the specification of educational, licensing, and clinical-experience requirements of practitioners, it is appropriate to identify and examine other components of a modern quality-management system to assess whether and under what circumstances counselors could serve as independent providers. The material in this chapter thus addresses determinants of high-quality mental health care for all mental health professionals at a clinical and systems level.

Several previous Institute of Medicine (IOM) reports on health-care quality, mental health and substance-abuse care, and treatment of posttraumatic stress disorder (PTSD) were especially influential in the committee's deliberations. In particular, the aims, rules, and frameworks set forth in *Crossing the Quality Chasm: A New Health System for the 21st Century* (IOM, 2001) provide an approach for this chapter and are summarized in the first section. The chapter then examines quality-of-care issues from clinical and systems perspectives and concludes with an examination of barriers to the implementation of clinical and systems strategies.

Appendix C contains the committee's working definitions of several key terms used in this chapter, including *diagnosis*, *treatment*, *psychotherapy*, and *quality*.

## GENERAL CONCEPTS OF HEALTH-CARE QUALITY AND "EVIDENCE-BASED PRACTICE"

### Health-Care Quality

Avedis Donabedian articulated as early as the 1960s a conceptual model for measuring health-care quality that remains highly relevant today. The model assesses three main components of health-care quality: structure, process, and outcome (Donabedian, 1966). *Structure* refers to characteristics of the health-care system or provider, such as training or clinic resources adequate for serving the population. *Process* refers to the care that is delivered—assessments, tests, and treatments. *Outcome* refers to the health status of patients after they receive care. Access to care and patient satisfaction are other important components of health-care quality (Donabedian, 1998).

Although it is desirable to know whether the care that is delivered to patients produces good outcomes, many factors that are independent of treatment quality can also affect a person's health status after treatment, including illness severity and the patient's ability and desire to adhere to a treatment regimen. Process measures of care, if they have a demonstrated link with outcomes, can therefore be useful tools for measuring treatment quality.

In the late 1990s, evidence, largely from research in processes of care, that health-care quality in America had serious and pervasive problems was mounting. Examples were inadequate access to care, unacceptable rates of medical errors, and patients receiving care that was not needed or not receiving care that was needed. IOM's Committee on the Quality of Health Care in America identified several underlying causes of the problems: the growing complexity of science and technology, which made it increasingly difficult for clinicians to stay abreast of new information; the shift from an acute-disease management paradigm to increasing management of chronic conditions; poor organization of the health-care system to meet the demands of the growing complexity and the paradigm shift; and inadequate use of information technology (IOM, 2001).

An IOM committee defined *quality* as "the degree to which health services for individuals and populations increase the likelihood of desired health outcomes and are consistent with current professional knowledge" (IOM, 1990, p. 4). Good quality means providing patients with services in a technically competent manner with good communication, shared decision making, and cultural sensitivity. *Crossing the Quality Chasm* laid the groundwork for a quality-driven approach to health care by adopting six aims governed by 10 rules as universal guidance for changes in the system and in provider–patient interactions. These are delineated in Tables 5.1 and 5.2, respectively.

Berwick (2002) noted that the report provided an underlying framework for the changes needed in American health care at four levels:

- Level A: the experience of patients.
- Level B: the functioning of small units of care delivery ("microsystems" such as a cardiac surgical team).
- Level C: the functioning of organizations that house or support microsystems (such as clinics and hospitals).
- Level D: the environment of policy, payment, regulation, accreditation, and other factors that influence the organization at Level C.

**TABLE 5.1** Aims of the Future Health-Care System

1. Safe—avoiding injuries to patients from the care that is intended to help them.
2. Effective—providing services based on scientific knowledge to all who could benefit and refraining from providing services to those not likely to benefit (avoiding underuse and overuse, respectively).
3. Patient-centered—providing care that is respectful of and responsive to individual patient preferences, needs, and values and ensuring that patient values guide all clinical decisions.
4. Timely—reducing waits and sometimes harmful delays for both those who receive and those who give care.
5. Efficient—avoiding waste, including waste of equipment, supplies, ideas, and energy.
6. Equitable—providing care that does not vary in quality because of personal characteristics such as gender, ethnicity, geographic location, and socioeconomic status.

SOURCE: IOM (2001).

**TABLE 5.2** Rules to Guide the Transition to a Health-Care System That Better Meets Patients' Needs

1. Care based on continuous healing relationships. Patients should receive care whenever they need it and in many forms, not just face-to-face visits. This rule implies that the health care system should be responsive at all times (24 hours a day, every day) and that access to care should be provided over the Internet, by telephone, and by other means in addition to face-to-face visits.
2. Customization based on patient needs and values. The system of care should be designed to meet the most common types of needs but have the capability to respond to individual patient choices and preferences.
3. The patient as the source of control. Patients should be given the necessary information and the opportunity to exercise the degree of control they choose over health care decisions that affect them. The health system should be able to accommodate differences in patient preferences and encourage shared decision making.
4. Shared knowledge and the free flow of information. Patients should have unfettered access to their own medical information and to clinical knowledge. Clinicians and patients should communicate effectively and share information.
5. Evidence-based decision making. Patients should receive care based on the best available scientific knowledge. Care should not vary illogically from clinician to clinician or from place to place.
6. Safety as a system property. Patients should be safe from injury caused by the care system. Reducing risk and ensuring safety require greater attention to systems that help prevent and mitigate errors.
7. The need for transparency. The health care system should make information available to patients and their families that allows them to make informed decisions when selecting a health plan, hospital, or clinical practice, or choosing among alternative treatments. This should include information describing the system's performance on safety, evidence-based practice, and patient satisfaction.
8. Anticipation of needs. The health system should anticipate patient needs, rather than simply reacting to events.
9. Continuous decrease in waste. The health system should not waste resources or patient time.
10. Cooperation among clinicians. Clinicians and institutions should actively collaborate and communicate to ensure an appropriate exchange of information and coordination of care.

SOURCE: IOM (2001), pp. 8-9.

It is critical that efforts to establish and improve quality address all levels with a central focus on affecting Level A—the experience of patients. Any committee recommendations regarding modifications of

TRICARE's policy on the practice of licensed mental health counselors should reflect the goals articulated in this framework.

*Crossing the Quality Chasm* called for

> purchasers, regulators, health professions, educational institutions and the Department of Health and Human Services [to] create an environment that fosters and rewards improvement by 1) creating an infrastructure to support evidence-based practice, 2) facilitating the use of information technology, 3) aligning payment incentives, and 4) preparing the work force to better serve patients in a world of expanding knowledge and rapid change. (IOM, 2001, p. 5)

That agenda applies directly to the role of TRICARE, its contractors, and mental health professions and organizations that serve the beneficiary population.

## Evidence-Based Practice

Achieving the changes described above requires a conceptual framework that uses both a clinical approach and a systems approach to delivering high-quality health care. In this framework, the practice of health care is designed so that each member of the clinical team has a defined role (e.g., physicians focus on acute-care delivery and patients who have not responded to treatment, and nonphysician clinicians focus on supporting chronic-care management that includes supporting patient self-management and follow-up); patients receive education about their illnesses and how to participate fully in their treatment, including self-monitoring of symptoms and behavioral change; clinicians receive continuing education and, when needed, clinical consultation; and clinicians have an information-support system that can provide reminders, monitor patient outcomes, provide feedback, and assist in treatment planning (Wagner et al., 1996).

The shift toward a systems approach to a high-quality infrastructure requires attention to more than the delivery of specific treatments. Nonetheless, evidence-based practice is an important part of the conceptual framework. The goal of evidence-based practice is to improve health-care quality by bringing to the usual practice the knowledge gained by clinical research (IOM, 2001, 2006; President's New Freedom Commission on Mental Health, 2002). Evidence-based practice applies the *best research evidence* combined with *clinical expertise* according to individual *patient values* (IOM, 2001). The best research evidence is obtained from clinical research and includes research in epidemiology, diagnosis, and treatment. Clinical expertise is gained from clinicians' training and experience in working with patients. Experience allows clinicians to be thoughtful, efficient, and accurate in providing patient care. It also enables them to provide compassionate care, which takes patients' values, preferences, and rights into account (Sackett et al., 1996).

High-quality care for mental and substance-use (M/SU)[1] conditions has several important components that are independent of the specific diagnosis for which a patient is treated. Clinicians who treat patients with M/SU conditions need to have adequate training. At the outset of treatment, M/SU clinicians need to be able to conduct a thorough clinical evaluation so that they can formulate a diagnosis and develop a treatment plan. Components of the evaluation include reasons for the evaluation; history of the presenting problem; past experiences with M/SU symptoms, behaviors, and treatment; medical history; information about family relationships and history of M/SU illnesses; developmental history; history of interpersonal functioning (family, friends, and work); legal history; a safety assessment that examines whether the patient or others are at risk of harm; and a mental-status examination to assess the patient's mood state, cognitive processes, and ability to function. Evaluations should include collateral information when possible, such as information from other clinicians, family members, or significant others and results of diagnostic medical tests and evaluations that might be used to exclude medical conditions that are causing or exacerbating symptoms. Clinicians need to determine, on the basis of the above evaluation, the appropriate treatment setting for the patient, such as inpatient versus outpatient (APA, 2006a). It is also important for clinicians to establish a therapeutic alliance with a patient at the outset of treatment to promote the patient's engagement and adherence, and to educate the patient and his or her family members about the condition for which the patient is being treated and about how to prevent or minimize exacerbations. Continuing tasks for M/SU clinicians include monitoring of a patient's response to treatment, assessing

[1]This chapter follows the convention of abbreviating "mental and substance-use" as "M/SU" established in IOM's *Improving the Quality of Health Care for Mental and Substance-Use Conditions* (2006).

function and safety, maintaining a therapeutic alliance, and monitoring and enhancing adherence. Systematic monitoring of patient response to treatment with established clinical scales and measures can improve M/SU outcomes, reducing symptoms and possibly avoiding hospitalization (Slade et al., 2006; Trivedi et al., 2006). Many patients who have M/SU conditions have co-occurring medical or other M/SU conditions, and integrating and coordinating treatment provided by multiple clinicians can be critical.

Once there is a diagnosis, clinicians must determine the most appropriate treatment for an individual patient on the basis of the clinical literature. Randomized controlled trials are an important part of the evidence base for understanding the efficacy of clinical treatments, but they are not the only evidence considered in evidence-based care. Often, patients enrolled in randomized controlled trials can differ substantially from those seen in usual care settings. For many patients and clinical scenarios, evidence from randomized controlled trials is sparse or nonexistent. Observational, nonrandomized studies can provide useful information about patients not typically seen in clinical trials. However, they may be subject to biases, and evidence-based practice requires an ability to evaluate a study systematically to determine whether it is valid in its conclusions and whether it is applicable to an individual patient (Evidence Based Medicine Working Group, 1992).

A barrier to implementing evidence-based practice is that not all clinicians have the appropriate training or adequate time to search the clinical literature independently and repeatedly to obtain the best, most recent evidence and to appraise it critically for validity and applicability. A survey of graduate psychotherapy training in psychiatry, psychology, and social work by Weissman and colleagues (2006) found that programs "often did not require the gold standard of didactic and clinical supervision for [evidence-based training]." Mullen et al. (2007), writing about social work professionals, cite several barriers to facilitating evidence-based training of current practitioners, including a nonsupportive workplace culture, infrastructure that does not provide the time and resources needed to access up-to-date best practices information, and limited resources to support the implementation of practices once they are identified.

There are resources, however, that can assist clinicians in implementing evidence-based care (Guyatt et al., 2000); such resources include reviews and guidelines that systematically review the literature and weigh the strength of evidence. Guidelines and systematic reviews, although useful in implementing evidence-based practices, have their own limitations. For example, they are not available for all clinical circumstances, and research evidence continues to evolve after a guideline or review is researched and published. Therefore, such resources should not be seen as a replacement for a practitioner's independent inquiry and critique of the diagnostic and treatment literature (Guyatt et al., 2000).

The RAND study described in Chapter 1 found that in the TRICARE population, the most prevalent diagnoses encountered by mental health and general medical clinicians are mood disorders, anxiety disorders, substance-use disorders, and adjustment disorders (Meredith et al., 2005). Many beneficiaries presented with co-occurring or multiple disorders. Although some TRICARE beneficiaries may need subspecialized mental health expertise to be treated for mental health conditions related to deployment and active combat, others can be well served by evidence-based practices available to the general population. Evidence-based guidelines exist to assist practitioners in accurate screening, diagnosis, and pharmacologic and psychosocial treatments for many of the conditions seen in the beneficiary population.

Table 5.3 provides examples of existing evidence-based psychosocial treatments for a sample of M/SU conditions that were either highlighted by TRICARE as conditions of particular interest or found to be among the more prevalent in the RAND study. Chapter 2 provides background information on them, briefly summarizing their signs and symptoms and their incidence rates. If an M/SU clinician is to conduct evidence-based practice, he or she needs to have training and experience in those treatments and have the capacity to learn and adapt as the evidence base on existing and new treatments expands. It is important to note that the table does not encompass all the evidence-based models for the conditions. Following the National Guideline Clearinghouse (2009) criteria for inclusion of clinical practice guidelines (CPGs), the table includes expert guidelines that are no more than 5 years old.[2] However, evidence-based practice continually evolves, so even guidelines that have been available for no more than 5 years can be outdated and not reflect the most recent literature. It is important to note that evidence-based medication treatment is available for each of the conditions in the

---

[2]That is, guidelines that were released no earlier than 2004 (the present report was written in 2009).

**TABLE 5.3** Examples of Evidence-Based Psychosocial Interventions for Selected Disorders Relevant to the TRICARE Beneficiary Population

| Disorder | Guideline-Recommended Treatment |
|---|---|
| Major depressive disorder | Cognitive behavioral therapy (APA, 2000; VA/DOD, 2009a)<br>Interpersonal therapy (VA/DOD, 2009a)<br>Dialectical behavioral therapy (VA/DOD, 2009a)<br>Behavioral couple therapy (VA/DOD, 2009a)<br>Problem-solving therapy (APA, 2005b; VA/DOD, 2009a) |
| Schizophrenia | Cognitive behavioral therapy (APA, 2004b; NIMH, 2009d)<br>Social-skills training (APA, 2004b)<br>Family intervention (APA, 2004b; NIMH, 2009d)<br>Assertive community treatment (APA, 2004b)<br>Supported employment (APA, 2004b; Lehman et al., 2004; NIMH, 2009d) |
| Acute stress disorder, posttraumatic stress disorder | Cognitive behavioral therapy (APA, 2004a, 2009a; NIMH, 2009c; VA/DOD, 2004)<br>Exposure therapy (APA, 2004a, 2009a; IOM, 2008; NIMH, 2009c; VA/DOD, 2004)<br>Eye-movement desensitization and reprocessing (APA, 2004a; VA/DOD, 2004) |
| Bipolar disorder | Cognitive behavioral therapy (APA, 2002, 2005a; NIMH, 2009b)<br>Interpersonal therapy (APA, 2002, 2005a; NIMH, 2009b)<br>Family-focused therapy (APA, 2002, 2005a; NIMH, 2009b) |
| Substance-use disorders | Cognitive behavioral therapy (APA, 2006b)<br>Motivational interviewing (APA, 2006b; VA/DOD, 2009b)<br>Behavioral couple therapy (APA, 2006b; VA/DOD, 2009b)<br>Cognitive behavioral skills training (VA/DOD, 2009b)<br>Contingency management (APA, 2006b; VA/DOD, 2009b)<br>Community reinforcement approach (APA, 2006b; VA/DOD, 2009b) |
| Generalized anxiety disorder | Cognitive behavioral therapy (DH, 2001; NIMH, 2009a)[a] |
| Obsessive-compulsive disorder | Exposure-response prevention (APA, 2007; Hill, 2007) |
| Panic disorder | Cognitive behavioral therapy (APA, 2009b) |

[a]The committee was not able to find American Psychiatric Association, Department of Veterans Affairs, or Department of Defense practice guidelines for generalized anxiety disorder.

table. For some conditions, such as bipolar disorder and schizophrenia, evidence-based practice recommends that patients receive medication to minimize symptoms or prevent repeated episodes of illness. For others—such as major depression, substance-use disorders, and anxiety disorders—medications can be efficacious, but patients who have symptoms or exacerbations may also be adequately treated with psychosocial interventions alone. Many patients can benefit from a combination of medication and psychosocial treatment.

## EVIDENCE-BASED PRACTICE FOR PSYCHOSOCIAL INTERVENTIONS TO ADDRESS CLINICAL ISSUES OF SPECIAL RELEVANCE TO THE TRICARE POPULATION

As noted above, the diagnoses and combinations of diagnoses for which TRICARE beneficiaries receive mental health care are quite varied. Evidence-based guidelines and systematic reviews do not exist for all of them. Even the guidelines that do exist may not apply fully or directly to people who are seeking care. Patients may manifest varying patterns of comorbidity (such as depression and substance abuse and traumatic brain injury), have pressing psychosocial problems that are not well characterized in a simple diagnostic category (such as traumatic grief and sexual assault), or present with clinical problems related to particular issues encountered in military life, such as combat in Operation Enduring Freedom (OEF) or Operation Iraqi Freedom (OIF). Therefore, clinicians must be able to monitor the scientific literature to adapt and adopt promising practices to fill gaps in available guidelines. This section describes examples of particular psychosocial interventions that, although not based on extensive evidence or formally recommended in guidelines, have been studied with regard to the particular needs of subsets of TRICARE beneficiaries.

Several central points should be considered. First, because most of the evidence-based practice models applicable to these issues are focused on remediation and symptom relief for the individual service member, it is important to be mindful of the synergistic effects of individual mental health issues in the context of the couple and family. This section therefore discusses clinical approaches that focus on individual, couple, and family issues.

Second, education in specific skills might be conflated with the ability to deliver high-quality care. Several researchers have warned about the danger of focusing too exclusively on operationalizing goals and interventions while sacrificing clinical skills that involve relational capacities, alliance building, and an ability to hold the complexity of the "client in social context" (Stein and Lambert, 1995).

Third, some guiding principles are useful in treating recently returned OIF or OEF service members, including these: establish a facilitative helping context that reduces stigma, facilitate family transitions and reduce conflict, prevent social isolation and withdrawal, support employment productivity, and prevent alcohol and other drug misuse and abuse (Ruzek et al., 2004).

The following subsections discuss various clinical intervention methods that have undergone some empirical study for assisting active-duty service members and their families with their mental health and psychosocial issues. The intent of this material is to illustrate the array of therapies available to clinicians for some conditions, not to be comprehensive. Mention of a particular therapy should not be viewed as an endorsement of its use in the TRICARE beneficiary population.

## Posttraumatic Stress Disorder

Several treatment models that address symptoms, affect regulation, and beliefs related to PTSD are oriented to not only the individual service member but partners, children, and other family members.

Treatment approaches include group, couple, and family therapy. Group therapy may focus on rebuilding connections and dealing with trauma-related rage, anger, guilt, and fear (Kingsley, 2007). Couple therapy and family therapy are often useful in educating family members about posttraumatic stress and PTSD responses, promoting communication, strengthening affect regulation, and facilitating new transitions (Harkness and Kador, 2001).

One cognitive-behavioral model specifically focuses on couples in which one partner is an OIF or OEF veteran who has a diagnosis of PTSD. Although the researchers are formally evaluating cognitive-behavioral couple therapy with such couples, they have been using the treatment for some time. The couples appear to benefit, as evidenced by increased relationship satisfaction, but most require more than the expected 15 sessions (Monson et al., 2008). One of the couple-therapy models, emotionally focused couple therapy (EFCT), designed by Susan Johnson as reported in Snyder et al. (2006), reportedly has strong empirical validation. It sustains an experiential, intrapsychic focus on attachment-based themes with an emphasis on interrupting destructive cyclic relational patterns. In four randomized trials, EFCT was superior to a waiting-list control condition in reducing relationship distress and yielded recovery rates of 70–73% and a weighted mean effect size of 1.31.

In addition to psychotherapy models that aim to remediate psychopathologic symptoms of covarying diagnoses, other evidence-based approaches focus on prevention and are important models for clinicians to understand and apply. For example, "battlemind training" was developed originally by Carl Castro and his colleagues at the Walter Reed Army Institute of Research and the US Army Medical Research and Materiel Command, who describe the model as evidence-based, explanatory, and focused on strengths rather than weaknesses. Building resilience is a major goal for service members, partners, and clinicians during the predeployment, deployment, and postdeployment phases of the deployment cycle. Rigorous studies that conducted training with a randomized controlled design led to data that suggested that soldiers who receive battlemind training reported fewer PTSD symptoms after deployment than soldiers who received the standard stress-education training. Studies suggest that battlemind training affects solders beyond the 1-hour training period by giving them the vocabulary to talk about mental health issues and normalize their symptoms and reactions. When the entire unit was trained together, members were more likely to talk with each other about their concerns (Castro, 2009; Surgeon General Multinational Force-Iraq, 2006).

The 2004 *VA/DOD Clinical Practice Guideline for PTSD* identified one pharmacotherapy—selective serotonin reuptake inhibitors (SSRIs)—and four psychotherapy interventions (cognitive therapy, exposure therapy, stress inoculation training, and eye-movement desensitization and reprocessing) as having "significant benefit" and an accompanying "strong recommendation that the intervention is always indicated and acceptable." A later IOM report on PTSD treatment (IOM, 2008) found that evidence from randomized controlled trials was sufficient to conclude that exposure therapies were effective in the treatment of PTSD but inadequate to draw conclusions on other therapies.

It observed, more generally, that research on treatment of PTSD in US veterans is inadequate to answer questions about interventions.

### Military Sexual Assault

The consequences of sexual harassment and assault can be complex and severe, including PTSD, but a variety of treatments can substantially reduce psychological symptoms and improve a victim's quality of life. There is little empirically based information on the treatment of sexual trauma associated with military service. However, extensive information is available on the treatment of civilian populations and can be used to inform treatment of active-duty and veteran populations. Interventions often address health and safety concerns; crisis intervention that provides normalizing posttrauma reactions; education about trauma; validation; support for existing coping and developing new modes of coping, including deep-breathing methods; and affective and cognitive reactions that include fear, self-blame, anger, and disillusionment. Brief psychodynamic therapy (Leichsenring et al., 2004), a form of cognitive restructuring (Foa and Rothbaum, 1998), and cognitive processing therapy (Resick and Schnicke, 2002) are useful treatment interventions. Again, including the partner in couple therapy is important in reducing shame and promoting more open communication.

### Depression with Suicidal Ideation or Behavior

Because traumatic grief is related most directly to the population of OEF and OIF service members, the phenomenon is briefly discussed here. *Traumatic grief* refers to the sudden loss of an important and close attachment. Having lost a close buddy and experiencing multiple losses often bring on immediate or prolonged grief. Survivor guilt, feelings of anger toward others who are thought to have caused the death, not being able to show vulnerability, numbing, and the absence of an opportunity in the field to acknowledge the death all contribute to unresolved grief. If grief symptoms persist beyond 6 months after return home, the service member may experience complicated grief. Clinical experience suggests the importance of recognizing the significance of the loss, restructuring distorted thoughts of guilt, and validating the pain and intensity of the feelings. There are no outcome studies of treatment for veterans for prolonged or complicated grief. When it is accompanied by a diagnosis of acute stress disorder or posttraumatic stress, cognitive therapy might be contraindicated because exposure to memories of traumatic events may cause a soldier even more strain (Jacobs and Prigerson, 2000). In each of those situations, involvement of the partner and other family members can provide necessary social support (IOM, 2008).

VA and DOD released a CPG for the management of major depressive disorder in 2009 (VA/DOD, 2009b). It recommended that cognitive behavioral therapy, interpersonal psychotherapy, and problem-solving therapy be used for the treatment of uncomplicated major depression, classifying the evidence supporting the recommendation as "A"—"good evidence was found that the intervention improves important health outcomes and . . . that benefits substantially outweigh harm." Other psychotherapies were identified as treatment options for specific populations or where indicated, based on patient preference. The guideline did not find sufficient evidence to recommend one antidepressant medication over another for all patients, and stated that the choice of medication should be based on "side effect profiles . . . , history of prior response, family history of response, type of depression, concurrent medical illnesses, concurrently prescribed medications, and cost of medication."

## Substance-Use Disorder

An evidence-based model titled Seeking Safety addresses the complex interaction of trauma-related issues and substance-use disorder (Najavits, 2007). It is one of the few models that focus on the intersection of covarying conditions, and it holds promise for service members who have suffered combat exposure and turn to substances of abuse, especially alcohol. For many of them, the misuse transforms into abuse or addiction. Treatment for substance abuse is enhanced by adjunctive couple or family therapy with involved family members.

The VA/DOD substance-use disorder CPG (VA/DOD, 2009c) recognizes behavioral couple therapy, cognitive behavioral coping skills training, motivational enhancement therapy, community reinforcement approach, and twelve-step facilitation as "first line alternatives at least as effective as other bona fide active interventions or treatment as usual" for at least some disorders. It recommended that motivational interviewing be used no matter which psychosocial intervention was employed.

## Traumatic Brain Injury

Active-duty service members may suffer traumatic brain injury (TBI) ranging in severity from mild to severe. In one study, only 47% of the troops who had a TBI met with a physician to assess the nature of the condition (Hoge et al., 2008). Symptoms of mild TBI (such as affect dysregulation, irritability, and sleep problems) often mirror the symptom picture of PTSD. After careful assessment with a thorough differential diagnosis, many service members are treated in rehabilitation settings. Treatment approaches may include cognitive rehabilitation with occupational and physical therapy to address the full array of general medical, cognitive, psychological, and psychosocial issues. Mental health approaches are also indicated to ease the transition of adjusting to temporary or permanent disabilities. Supportive, relationally based methods that stress the reparative nature of a positive therapeutic alliance are preferable during the period when the client's cognitive functioning is impaired. Couple and family therapy methods can help partners and children to understand the effects of polytrauma, defined as damage to more than one organ system (e.g., TBI, hearing loss, amputations, visual impairment, and burns).

The VA/DOD CPG for the management of concussion and mild TBI (VA/DOD, 2009a) indicated that patients be screened for psychiatric symptoms and comorbid psychiatric disorders, specifically mentioning depression, posttraumatic stress, and substance use. It recommended that "[t]reatment of psychiatric/behavioral symptoms following concussion/mTBI should be based upon individual factors and nature and severity of symptom presentation, and include both psychotherapeutic [Strength of Recommendation (SR) = A] and pharmacological [SR = I][3] treatment modalities."

[3]The Guideline defines a Strength of Recommendation (SR) = A as "[a] strong recommendation that the clinicians provide the intervention to eligible patients. Good evidence was found that the intervention improves important health outcomes and concludes that benefits substantially outweigh harm." An SR = I means that "[t]he conclusion is that the evidence is insufficient to recommend for or against routinely providing the intervention. Evidence that the intervention is effective is lacking, or poor quality, or conflicting, and the balance of benefits and harms cannot be determined."

## EMPIRICAL EVIDENCE REGARDING DISTINCTIONS BETWEEN THE PRACTICE OF COUNSELORS AND THE PRACTICE OF OTHER MENTAL HEALTH PROFESSIONALS

The statement of task asked the committee to review outcome studies and the literature on the comparative quality and effectiveness of care provided by licensed mental health counselors. Despite an extensive review, the committee identified no literature bearing directly on that question. Research related to more general characteristics of mental health practitioners and the care delivered by them was found and is discussed below.

A small set of studies compared novice practitioners (typically graduate students) and experienced practitioners. Mayfield et al. (1999) found that graduate students in counseling psychology produced simpler, more hierarchic cognitive maps and required more time to process information than did practicing counselors who held doctoral degrees in that field. Kivlighan and Kivlighan (2009) analyzed knowledge structures of group-counseling trainees and found that, after taking a graduate-level group practicum class, their cognitive maps became more complex and hierarchic and more like those of experienced practitioners. Mallinckrodt and Nelson (1991) examined novice, advanced, and experienced practitioners' therapeutic alliances and found that counseling psychologists who had higher training levels were given higher client ratings for agreement on overall goals of treatment and tasks relevant to achieving the goals but not on emotional bonds between practitioner and client. Finally, Cummings et al. (1993) found that clients of experienced mental health services practitioners (three PhD psychologists and one advanced graduate student) rated sessions as deeper than did clients of novice practitioners, and experienced practitioners recalled different types of important events than novice practitioners. Experience was used as a proxy for expertise in those studies, and the researchers did not attempt to link differences in cognitive structures, working alliance, or session evaluation to differences in treatment effectiveness. Samples were small, and that might limit the generalizability of the results; and the definitions of *novice* and *experienced* were somewhat arbitrary and inconsistent among studies.

A number of meta-analyses and reviews have examined mental health therapy effectiveness, but they do not provide evidence on the comparative effectiveness of treatment by different types of mental health–care providers. Many of the studies grouped various types of mental health providers, often without explicitly including mental health counselors (e.g., Berman and Norton, 1985; Durlak, 1979; Seligman, 1995). Others examined levels of training or experience within a given discipline, typically psychology (McPherson et al., 2000; Spengler et al., 2009; Stein and Lambert, 1995). Some studies were based on practitioners in other countries (Bower and Rowland, 2006)—who have different education, training, and licensure standards from their US counterparts—or were conducted so long ago that their results are no longer relevant to professionals practicing now (Durlak, 1979; Smith and Glass, 1977). Finally, reviewers (Berman and Norton, 1985; Nietzel and Fisher, 1981) asserted that many studies suffered from methodologic flaws, such as inconsistency in defining professional status and improper statistical interpretation.

It can be argued that such systematic reviews yield indirect evidence of provider effectiveness. That at least some of the studies examined documented service provision by counselors with other mental health professionals might suggest that counselors—when provided, like other mental health professionals, with appropriate training and monitoring—can effectively provide evidence-based psychosocial interventions. It is clearly insufficient information on which to base conclusions about the effectiveness of care by any professional group, but it does indicate that each of the professions has the capacity to provide some types of effective evidence-based care under proper conditions.

Arguments of differential effectiveness by mental health–provider type—such as the statement by McPherson et al. (2000, p. 696) that "one would expect that [doctoral-level] psychologists would be better prepared to identify problems and errors with various types of psychological assessment data than would master's-level providers"—are generally not based on empirical evidence but are instead founded on anecdotal information or supposition. As Spengler et al. (2009, p. 353) noted, "there are no comprehensive quantitative analyses on . . . whether any form of educational experience is linked to clinical judgment accuracy."

## STRATEGIES FOR MONITORING AND IMPROVING THE QUALITY OF BEHAVIORAL HEALTH CARE

The IOM report *Improving the Quality of Health Care for Mental and Substance-Use Conditions* (2006) identified a series of problems in quality and reviewed various studies that documented discrepancies between care that is known to be effective and care that is actually delivered, and it reported extensive variations in care from provider to provider. The report also noted that the infrastructure needed to measure, analyze, publicly report, and improve the quality of M/SU health care is less well developed than that of general health care. Nonetheless, the report presented a blueprint for building the infrastructure for M/SU health care that has important implications for the provision of counseling and other mental health services for TRICARE beneficiaries.

## Strategies for Measuring the Quality of Care

Throughout the quality-improvement field, the general mantra has been that "you can't improve what you don't measure." The 2006 IOM report *Improving the Quality of Care* emphasized that effectively measuring quality requires structures, resources, and expertise and strategic efforts among key stakeholders to

- Conceptualize the aspects of care to be measured.
- Translate the quality-of-care measurement concepts into performance-measure specifications.
- Pilot-test the performance-measure specifications to determine their validity, reliability, feasibility, and cost.
- Ensure calculation of the performance measures and their submission to a performance-measure repository.
- Audit to ensure that the performance measures have been calculated accurately and in accordance with specifications.
- Analyze and display the performance measures in a format or formats suitable for understanding by multiple intended audiences, such as consumers, health-care–delivery entities, purchasers, and quality-oversight organizations.
- Maintain the effectiveness of individual performance measures and performance-measure sets and policies.

The IOM motto—a quote from Goethe—is "Knowing is not enough; we must apply. Willing is not enough; we must do." In that spirit, simply measuring quality is not enough; measurement is in the service of improving care at all four levels of the health-care system—

Levels A–D of Berwick (2002). A substantial literature documents effective strategies for improvement in industry generally, in general health care, and in M/SU health care.

A useful approach to applying quality-measurement and quality-improvement concepts to counseling and other psychosocial interventions in the Donabedian structure–process–outcomes model previously described is outlined below. From a structural point of view, one would want to incorporate measures in the following categories:

- Are providers trained in evidence-based practices (as incorporated in certification, credentialing, and licensing)?
- Are providers trained in applying evidence-based practices to different M/SU conditions and developing competences?
- Do clinicians or organized care settings have mechanisms to ensure that patients are receiving evidence-based care and use mechanisms to measure and improve the quality of care (e.g., as incorporated in provider agreements with TRICARE contractors)?
- Do care providers have mechanisms to measure, evaluate, and improve the quality of care (including the provision of evidence-based care) of their providers and contractors and for the population to be served?

Process measures might include the following categories:

- Are providers using evidence-based practices as applied to assessment, diagnosis, and treatment
  —At a level of fidelity that meets accepted standards?
  —Of all disorders or conditions presenting in the treatment setting?
  —By mental health–clinician category?
- Are clinics and other organized settings using the mechanisms to assess whether patients are receiving evidence-based care and using the data to improve care?
- Are care contractors using the mechanisms to assess whether patients are receiving evidence-based care and using the data to improve the performance of providers in their network?

Finally, from an outcomes perspective:

- Are providers, clinics, and care contractors systematically gathering appropriate measures of clinical outcomes and using the data to improve outcomes of their patients and populations?
- Are the outcomes improving?

### Systems Approaches for Monitoring and Improving Interventions

Evidenced-based treatments available for some common M/SU conditions vary and multiple psychotherapeutic approaches are used to treat people for the same condition. Some appropriate variation in treatment approaches is expected to align with the aims and rules outlined by *Crossing the Quality Chasm: A New Health System for the 21st Century* (IOM, 2001) when based on the specific needs that patients bring to the therapeutic setting. Patients presents with symptoms of a condition that support a diagnosis, but the effectiveness of patient treatment is heavily influenced by myriad other factors, such as ability to establish a therapeutic alliance, patient acceptance and motivation to change, cognitive ability to participate in therapy, and ability to learn and improve adaptive skills and generalize the new skills outside the therapeutic setting.

Despite substantial evidence of the efficacy of numerous treatments for M/SU problems and illnesses, treatments delivered in practice—like all health care—often are not consistent with evidence-based practices or consensus guidelines (IOM, 2006), nor are evidenced-based treatments delivered with the same degree of fidelity among therapists. Variation in behavioral health care is driven by a variety of factors, some germane to the structure and process of the behavioral health–service delivery system and others individualized to the needs of patients. Variance to meet the needs of patients is consistent with one of the *Crossing the Quality Chasm* aims and rules. It is appropriate for trained clinicians to tailor therapeutic regimens to patients' unique clinical conditions, relevant environmental factors, and patients' adaptive, cognitive, and motivational levels and skills. Variance due to differences in training and acquired skills and to infidelity in the application of evidenced-based therapies that affect the ability to assess, diagnose, and treat patients effectively for health conditions is considered problematic and inconsistent with high-quality care.

Variability of care in behavioral health is confounded by the great variability in the behavioral health workforce in the delivery of nonpharmacologic treatments or interventions for M/SU conditions. The workforce includes licensed clinicians (state designation), certified (specialty societies), paraprofessionals, peers, and in some cases family members. As the present report makes clear, clinicians trained to diagnose and treat M/SU conditions are especially varied. Training in these disciplines differs widely and holds no assurance of exposure or of competence to treat all M/SU conditions. It thus recommends that institutions of higher education place a much greater emphasis on interdisciplinary didactic and experiential learning and bring together faculty and trainees from their various education programs in order to facilitate the development and implementation of core competencies across all M/SU disciplines. Chapter 3 notes that the ability to practice independently as determined by state statutes, boards of regulation and licensure, and various certifications does not require any demonstrations of competence in assessment, diagnosis, or treatment other than those stipulated by the individual training and graduation requirements of each discipline.

Variability in the clinical setting due to the variability from provider to provider is a serious problem. Research has consistently demonstrated that therapists vary in their effectiveness and that the therapist has a great influence on treatment outcomes (Blatt et al., 1996; Crits-Christoph et al., 1991; Luborsky et al., 1997; Project MATCH Research Group, 1998). Wampold and Brown (2005) estimated that ~5% of the variation in outcomes in a managed-care setting was attributable to variability between therapists. An earlier analysis by Wampold (2001) calculated that 1–2% of that variance was due to the type of treatment delivered. The variability among therapists becomes greater as the initial severity of a patient's illness increases (Kim et al., 2006). In practice settings, some psychotherapists consistently attain better outcomes than others, and this seems to be true regardless of patient diagnoses, age, developmental stage, medication status, and severity—good therapists get consistently better outcomes in a wide array of patients (Wampold and Brown, 2005).

The therapeutic alliance has been conceptualized over the years as an important part of the "glue" that keeps patients in treatment and perhaps explains some of the large differences among therapists beyond differences in training in evidenced-based treatments. Studies have demonstrated that the therapeutic alliance has a substantial effect on and correlation with treatment outcome (Wampold, 2001). The therapeutic alliance has been defined by Bordin (1979) as consisting of mutual construction of a goal shared by patient and therapist, accepted recognition of the task that each person is to perform in the relationship, and the presence of an attachment bond. The question has been whether developing a therapeutic alliance with one's patients is a skill acquired through training or a personality trait. Over the years, research and training programs have evolved curricula and techniques to enhance a therapist's ability to be aware of and introduce into the therapeutic setting the building blocks for development (Grace et al., 1995; Lambert et al., 2005; Mallinckrodt and Nelson, 1991; Weiden and Havens, 1994). In a review of that research involving psychologists and counselors, Summers and Barber (2003) concluded that the ability to develop a therapeutic alliance can be developed during training and may improve through acquisition of specific skills, accumulated hours of clinical practice, and more complex case conceptualization. Trainees become more focused on the therapeutic alliance with greater training and clinical experience, but some aspects of the alliance, such as goal setting and task recognition, may be more learnable and teachable than bond development. One important factor is preexisting aspects of a therapist's personality, which can affect the ability to develop a therapeutic bond. Development of an effective therapeutic alliance does not depend on provider discipline.

With the demonstration of the effectiveness of evidenced-based treatments, delivery of behavioral health treatments with fidelity is important. Treatment fidelity refers to the methodologic strategies used to monitor and enhance the reliability and consistency of clinical services. Consistent psychosocial therapy is more of a challenge than consistent medication, of which Food and Drug Administration requirements ensure the consistency of dosing and ingredients. The goal for therapeutic approaches is to reach a level of accuracy or consistency that is reproducible in each appropriate clinical case and results in the same outcomes in a population of like subjects.

Recognition that there is variability among individual therapists' techniques and that the therapist has a substantial effect on treatment outcomes points to a need to identify methods to ensure that psychosocial therapies are delivered with fidelity. In research settings where behavioral-change interventions are a part of the design, there is a great need for fidelity. A National Institutes of Health (NIH) workgroup was formed—the Treatment Fidelity Workgroup of the NIH Behavior Change Consortium (BCC)—to identify best practices and recommendations for enhancing the fidelity of behavioral-change interventions (Bellg et al., 2004). The degree of rigor required in research to ensure fidelity is not the same as for clinical practice, but the recommendations from the workgroup are still relevant and outline useful structure and process procedures that can be applied to assessing the quality of providers.

The best practices and recommendations from the BCC consist of the four domains—provider training, delivery of treatment, receipt of treatment, and enactment of treatment skills—and goals for each domain and recommended strategies to achieve them (Table 5.4).

Consistent strategies for improving the fidelity of psychosocial therapies among domains included use of standardized training materials in a manualized format with scripting, video or audio monitoring of intervention periodically by supervisors during and after training, and use of measurement and feedback with the provider and patient. The BCC concluded that the implementation of therapies needs to be evaluated and monitored on an individual basis during the training period and after training is over to prevent drift in skills. Another important conclusion was that measurement and monitoring of patient response (understanding of the intervention and demonstration of response) by the provider is important to reinforce and build treatment fidelity. While many of the recommendations are a part of the structure and process of provider training programs, posttraining systems to reinforce treatment fidelity and prevent a drift in skills are limited. Posttraining providers may be required to demonstrate attendance at and knowledge gained from educational sessions to maintain licensure or certification.

Systems to measure treatment outcome are in place as a part of accreditation of health plans (the National Committee for Quality Assurance and URAC) and delivery systems (the Joint Commission and the Commission on Accreditation of Rehabilitation Facilities). Most focus on structure and process measurement on the basis of best-practice guidelines and systems rather than individual providers. Health plans, hospitals, and accredited clinics and facilities—through their credentialing and recredentialing, their privileging processes, and their continuing monitoring of provider performance through complaints, sentinel events, and satisfaction—have the best view of provider performance

**TABLE 5.4** National Institutes of Health Behavior Change Consortium Best-Practice Domains and Recommendations

| Domain | Goal | Strategies |
|---|---|---|
| Provider training | Standardize training for all provider types | Standardized training manuals, materials, resources, field guides; structure practice and role-playing; use standardized patients; use same instructors, videotape training |
| | Ensure provider skill acquisition | Observe intervention implementation with standardized patient or role-playing; score provider according to checklist; conduct debriefing; administer written pretraining and posttraining examinations; certify skills during and after training |
| | Minimize "drift" in provider skills | Conduct booster sessions; conduct in vivo observations scored against checklist; supervise; obtain provider self-report; conduct patient exit interviews or otherwise obtain feedback |
| | Accommodate provider difference | Have professional supervise paraprofessional providers; monitor dropout rates, treatment effectiveness |
| Delivery of treatment | Control for provider difference | Assess patients' perception of provider via questionnaire, give feedback to provider; audiotape sessions, have different supervisors review; monitor patient complaints; have provider work with all treatment groups |
| | Reduce differences within treatment | Use scripted protocols, treatment manuals; have supervisors rate audiotapes, videotapes |
| | Ensure adherence to treatment protocol | Audiotape or videotape encounter, review with provider; randomly monitor audiotapes for protocol adherence; have provider complete checklist of intervention components |
| Receipt of treatment and enactment of treatment skills | Ensure patient comprehension | Have provider review participant homework, self-monitoring logs; have structured interview with patient |
| | Ensure patient ability to use cognitive skills | Have providers review homework; assess, measure participant performance; use questionnaires; use hypothetical scenarios to test patient |
| | Ensure patient ability to perform behavioral skills | Collect patient self-monitoring, self-report data; use behavioral-outcome measures |

SOURCE: Excerpted and adapted from Bellg et al. (2004).

after training but are aligned with only a few of the BCC recommendations for posttraining strategies.

The health-care professions are also moving toward a more comprehensive view of the means by which practitioners demonstrate that they have retained and updated the fund of knowledge and clinical skills that were initially recognized through the successful completion of training, examinations and licensure at the beginning of their careers. The American Board of Medical Specialties, which sets standards and processes for certifying and recertifying physicians, has adopted standards for mandatory "maintenance of certification" (MOC) programs that focus on professional standing, lifelong learning and self-assessment, cognitive expertise, and evaluation of performance in practice. Psychiatrists who obtained board certification after October 1994 are subject to a 10-year MOC program that will—when fully implemented in 2017—require diplomates to complete broad-based continuing self-assessment educational activities in addition to continuing medical education, an examination testing their knowledge of research developments and practice guidelines, and three rounds of chart and patient/peer reviews as conditions of recertification (ABPN, 2009). Diplomates in some psychiatric subspecialties are additionally required to demonstrate specific knowledge in their field. The 2010 IOM report *Redesigning Continuing Education in the Health Professions* noted:

> [The MOC] concept has not yet been adopted by all professions that grant certification. However, if minimum standards were applied across the health professions (given that different professions require different amounts of learning), the public could be ensured that all practitioners, despite their profession or specialty, have the ability to perform competently and to improve the safety and quality of health care. (pp. 134-135)

Systems that measure ongoing provider performance have been implemented. IOM's *Improving the Quality . . .* report noted (IOM, 2006, p. 160):

> In the Veterans Health Administration (VHA), linking outcome data on patients treated for posttraumatic stress disorder with administrative data showed that long-term, intensive inpatient treatment was not more effective than short-term treatment and cost $18,000 more per patient per year (Fontana and Rosenheck, 1997; Rosenheck and

> Fontana, 2001). In 1999, the VHA mandated that all mental health inpatients be rated at discharge using the GAF instrument,[4] and that all outpatients be similarly rated at least once every 90 days during active treatment. The agency now includes GAF outcome measures in its National Mental Health Program Performance Monitoring System (Greenberg and Rosenheck, 2005).

As a part of training and continuous development of therapeutic-alliance competences, Summers and Barber (2003) recommended that, as in clinical research settings, alliance should be rated repeatedly during therapy at sessions 2, 5, and 10 and every 3 months for longer periods of psychotherapy on at least three patients.

Lambert and colleagues (2005) reviewed four studies that evaluated the effect of clinical feedback systems in more than 2,500 cases. They consistently found that outcome feedback systems enhanced the outcome in patients who were not improving early in their treatment: 35% of patients whose therapists received outcome feedback improved in contrast with 21% of patients whose therapists did not receive feedback. Another study (Brown et al., 2001) examined the naturalistic effect of implementing an outcome feedback system in a managed-care outpatient network. The analysis, based on 15,000 cases, confirmed that patients whose therapists received feedback had more than 25% greater improvement than patients whose therapists did not receive feedback.

To assess the quality of behavioral health–care delivery in the TRICARE system, it would be important to use a working definition of *high-quality behavioral health care* that takes into account the six aims (Table 5.1) and 10 rules (Table 5.2) and—as identified through research and evidence—the key indicators of structure, process, and outcomes. The framework of a high-quality care system encompasses many factors:

- Use of effectively trained and certified providers in evidenced-based practices applied to specific populations and use of methods to ensure fidelity of technique.

---

[4]The Global Assessment of Functioning (GAF) score is a standardized measure of symptoms and psychosocial function in which 100 represents superior mental health and psychosocial function and 0 represents the worst possible state. The 2007 IOM report *PTSD Compensation and Military Service* contains a comprehensive review of the usefulness of GAF scores in evaluating PTSD.

—Use of well-trained supervisory systems based on the recommendations of the BCC.
—Use of objective outcome-measurement systems.
—Declaration of successful training by technique, conditions, and special populations.

- Use of postgraduation or postcertification continuous retraining techniques to ensure continued treatment effectiveness, fidelity, and training in new or enhanced treatment techniques as appropriate.
- Consistent use of evidence-based practices in diagnosis, assessment, and monitoring, supported by the use of validated instruments as an adjunct to clinical judgment.
- Use of an outcome-informed measurement system to support the effective application of treatment on an individual level and a systems level.

## BARRIERS TO IMPLEMENTING CLINICAL AND SYSTEMS QUALITY-IMPROVEMENT STRATEGIES

The ability of health-care organizations to put quality improvement mechanisms in place is limited by various barriers. Among the barriers identified in the 2006 *Improving the Quality* . . . report are the following:

1. Insufficient evidence or guidelines. There is strong evidence of the effectiveness of many treatments for M/SU conditions, but for many conditions, particularly in persons who have co-occurring disorders, there is inadequate evidence of effective treatments. These gaps in the knowledge base hinder the development of evidence-based guidelines for training and measurement.
2. Lack of standardized elements of care. The ability to measure quality of care depends heavily on access to the data necessary to document the provision of evidence-based care. Ideally, the information can be obtained inexpensively through administrative data, such as claims. However, current systems for coding psychological treatments are not refined enough to characterize the type of therapy or to document the degree of fidelity with which it is provided. Nevertheless, administrative and other elec-

tronic data can be useful in assisting clinicians and policy makers in measuring treatment quality.

3. Variability and lack of specificity of training, accreditation, certification, and licensing procedures that ensure an adequately prepared workforce that can provide evidence-based treatments.
4. Lack of adequate information systems to measure and monitor the quality of patient care, providers, practices, plans, and purchasers.

Government organizations—including the Department of Veterans Affairs and the Department of Health and Human Services Agency for Healthcare Research and Quality, the Centers for Medicare & Medicaid Services, NIH, and the Substance Abuse and Mental Health Services Administration—have been pursuing research and initiatives intended to overcome such barriers.

## QUALITY-OF-CARE INITIATIVES IN TRICARE AND THE MILITARY HEALTH SYSTEM

A thorough review of quality-of-care initiatives in TRICARE and the Military Health System (MHS) is beyond the scope of this report. This section briefly summarizes the results of some of the recent reports published on the topic by DOD and by organizations that were asked to perform work for it.

Health-care quality is identified as a key mission element of the MHS (TRICARE, 2009). In 2008, the Assistant Secretary of Defense for Health Affairs, testifying on mental health before a subcommittee of the House of Representatives Committee on Armed Services, stated that DOD's quality-of-care initiative "relies on developing and disseminating clinical guidance and standards, as well as training clinicians in clinical practice guidelines and effective evidence-based methods of care" (Casscells, 2008). DOD established the Defense Centers of Excellence for Psychological Health and Traumatic Brain Injury in late 2007 to lead the effort.

In response to a mandate contained in the National Defense Authorization Act for Fiscal Year 2007 (Public Law 109-364), DOD contracted for an independent review of its medical quality-improvement program, including efforts by TRICARE's purchased-care contractors. The resulting report (Lumetra, 2008, p. 2) concluded that "MHS quality and patient safety programs are generally comparable to those found in civilian facilities, and the MHS processes to establish criteria and measure quality are of high standard." The Lumetra study included a review of mental health quality issues. It reported that purchased-care contractors were critical of what they deemed an expensive and redundant federal requirement for dual certification of mental and behavioral health facilities but had no other specific comments.

Other reviews, however, have provided some details that highlighted quality concerns in the MHS. A directive contained in § 723 of the FY 2006 National Defense Authorization Act (Public Law 109-163) instructed DOD to convene a task force to assess mental health services provided by the MHS and to offer recommendations for improving their efficacy. The task force released its report, titled *An Achievable Vision*, in June 2007 (DOD Task Force on Mental Health, 2007). It noted (p. 33) that although the department had developed evidence-based CPGs for PTSD, depression, substance abuse, and psychosis,[5]

> these guidelines are not consistently implemented across the DOD and the Task Force was unable to find any mechanism that ensures their widespread use. Furthermore, providers who were interested in utilizing evidence-based approaches complained during site visits that they did not have the time to implement them.

It concluded (p. 20) that "DOD's mental health providers require additional training regarding current and new state-of-the-art practice guidelines."

The task force also found that there was "no consistent system for ongoing quality assessment and continuous improvement that includes substantial measurements of psychological health care outcomes" (p. 33). It concluded that "there are not sufficient mechanisms in place to assure the use of evidence-based treatments or the monitoring of treatment effectiveness" and that "the TRICARE network benefit for psychological health is hindered by fragmented rules and policies, inadequate oversight, and insufficient reimbursement" (p. ES-3).

Among the recommendations that were offered in reaction to those findings were two that addressed quality of care:

[5]DOD and VA later promulgated an additional CPG for TBI.

- 5.2.3.3: The Department of Defense should ensure that mental health professionals apply evidence-based clinical practice guidelines.
- 5.2.3.4: The Department of Defense should routinely track and analyze patient outcomes to ensure treatment efficacy.

In addition, the task force underscored the need for TRICARE providers to be specifically trained to meet the needs of their patient population:

- 5.3.4.9: The Department of Defense should improve TRICARE providers' training in issues related to military experiences by:
  - — Requiring that TRICARE mental health contractors offer mediated training packages to all network mental health providers similar to those available through the National Center for Post-Traumatic Stress Disorder, the Department of Defense Center for Deployment Psychology, and military mental health components.
  - — Requiring that TRICARE mental health contractors offer training packages for specific disorders and problems such as post-traumatic stress disorder and other combat stress syndromes each time a treatment plan is approved.

DOD published a response to the *Achievable Vision* report in September 2007, outlining the steps that it would take to implement the recommendations (DOD, 2007). The department pledged to emphasize the use of CPGs through a policy memorandum, to create and implement new CPGs, and to facilitate training in them. It also stated that it would review its outcome measures and policies, develop new evidence-based measures as needed, and issue directives requiring the use of outcome measures.

Separately, the DOD Inspector General's office generated observations and a critique of the task force's work (DOD Office of Inspector General, 2008). It echoed the conclusions regarding evidence-based treatments and indicated that health-care program managers "need to do more to monitor, oversee, and improve effectiveness."

## OBSERVATIONS

On the basis of the review of the papers, reports, and other information discussed in this chapter, the committee observes that

- The statutes and regulations under which TRICARE operates use educational, licensing, and clinical-experience requirements to determine the circumstances under which mental health professionals practice. That constitutes a system of quality management.
- The scientific literature on the delivery of health services—including mental health services—indicates that high-quality care is achieved through a patient-centered system grounded in the delivery of evidence-based clinical practices and the monitoring of outcomes.
- There are established clinical evidence-based practices endorsed by professional guidelines relevant to mental health care for the TRICARE population.
- There is a set of systems practices that are appropriate for monitoring and improving the quality of mental health care (including outcome measurement) and can be applied in the management of the TRICARE system.
- All providers should be prepared to deliver evidence-based practices in their scope of practice and to be trained in following and evaluating the accumulating evidence base with regard to promising treatments for problems that are particularly relevant to members of the military and their families.
- TRICARE and its contractors should implement effective systems-level quality-monitoring and quality-improvement practices.

## REFERENCES

ABPN (American Board of Psychiatry and Neurology). 2009. *The ABPN Maintenance of Certification (MOC) program* (rev. 07/26/09). http://www.abpn.com/downloads/moc/moc_web_doc.pdf. (Accessed December 10, 2009).

APA (American Psychiatric Association). 2000. *Practice guideline for the treatment of patients with major depressive disorder,* 2nd ed. Arlington, VA: APA.

APA. 2002. *Practice guideline for the treatment of patients with bipolar disorder,* 2nd ed. Arlington, VA: APA.

APA. 2004a. *Practice guideline for the treatment of patients with acute stress disorder and posttraumatic stress disorder.* Arlington, VA: APA.

APA. 2004b. *Practice guideline for the treatment of patients with schizophrenia,* 2nd ed. Arlington, VA: APA.

APA. 2005a. *Guideline watch: Practice guideline for the treatment of patients with bipolar disorder,* 2nd ed. Arlington, VA: APA.

APA. 2005b. *Guideline watch: Practice guideline for the treatment of patients with major depressive disorder,* 2nd ed. Arlington, VA: APA.

APA. 2006a. *Practice Guideline for the Psychiatric evaluation of adults,* 2nd ed. Arlington, VA: APA.

APA. 2006b. *Practice guideline for the treatment of patients with substance use disorders,* 2nd ed. Arlington, VA: APA.

APA. 2007. *Practice guideline for the treatment of patients with obsessive-compulsive disorder.* Arlington, VA: APA.

APA. 2009a. *Guideline watch: Practice guideline for the treatment of patients with acute stress disorder and posttraumatic stress disorder.* Arlington, VA: APA.

APA. 2009b. *Practice guideline for the treatment of patients with panic disorder.* Arlington, VA: American Psychiatric Publishing, Inc.

Bellg AJ, Borrelli B, Resnick B, Hecht J, Minicucci DS, Ory M, Ogedegbe G, Orwig D, Ernst D, Czajkowski, S. 2004. Enhancing treatment fidelity in health behavior change studies: Best practices and recommendations from the Behavior Change Consortium. *Health Psychology* 23(5):443-451.

Berman JS, Norton NC. 1985. Does professional training make a therapist more effective? *Psychological Bulletin* 98(2):401-407.

Berwick D. 2002. A user's manual for the IOM's "Quality chasm" report. *Health Affairs* 21(3):80-90.

Blatt SJ, Sanislow CA, Zuroff DC, Pilkonis PA. 1996. Characteristics of effective therapists: Further analyses of data from the National Institute of Mental Health Treatment of Depression Collaborative Research Program. *Journal of Consulting and Clinical Psychology* 64(6):1276-1284.

Bordin ES. 1979. The generalizability of the psychoanalytic concept of the working alliance. *Psychotherapy: Theory, Research, and Practice* 16(3):252-260.

Bower PJ, Rowland N. 2006. Effectiveness and cost effectiveness of counseling in primary care. *Cochrane Database of Systematic Reviews* 3(CD001025):1-75.

Brown GS, Burlingame GM, Lambert MJ, Jones E, Vaccaro J. 2001. Pushing the quality envelope: A new outcomes management system. *Psychiatric Services* 52(7):925-934.

Casscells SW. 2008. Statement on mental health by the Honorable S. Ward Casscells, MD, Assistant Secretary of Defense for Health Affairs before the Subcommittee on Military Personnel of the Armed Services Committee, U.S. House of Representatives, March 14. http://www.dod.mil/dodgc/olc/docs/testCasscells080314.pdf. (Accessed October 9, 2009).

Castro C. 2009. Impact of combat on the mental health and well-being of soldiers and marines. *Smith College Studies in Social Work* 79(3/4):249-264.

Crits-Christoph P, Baranackie K, Kurcias JS, Beck AT, Carroll K, Perry K, Luborsky L, McLellan A, Woody G, Thompson L, Gallagher D, Zitrin C. 1991. Meta-analysis of therapist effects in psychotherapy outcome studies. *Psychotherapy Research* 1(2):81-91.

Cummings AL, Slemon AG, Hallberg ET. 1993. Session evaluation and recall of important events as a function of counselor experience. *Journal of Counseling Psychology* 40(2):156-165.

DH (Department of Health). 2001. *Treatment choice in psychological therapies and counseling: Evidence based clinical practice guideline.* London: DH.

DOD (Department of Defense). 2007. *The Department of Defense plan to achieve the vision of the DOD Task Force on Mental Health: Report to Congress,* September. http://www.dcoe.health.mil/Content/Navigation/Documents/MHTF-Report-to-Congress.pdf. (Accessed October 8, 2009).

DOD Office of Inspector General. 2008. *Observations and critique of the DOD Task Force on Mental Health.* Report No. IE-2008-003, April 15. www.dodig.mil/Inspections/IE/Reports/IE-2008-003.pdf. (Accessed October 8, 2009).

DOD Task Force on Mental Health. 2007. *An achievable vision: Report of the Department of Defense Task Force on Mental Health.* Falls Church, VA: Defense Health Board. http://www.health.mil/dhb/mhtf/MHTF-Report-Final.pdf. (Accessed October 8, 2009).

Donabedian A. 1966. Evaluating the quality of medical care. *Milbank Quarterly* 44(3 Pt. 2):166-203.

Donabedian A. 1998. The quality of health care: how can it be assessed? *Journal of the American Medical Association* 260(12):1743-1748.

Durlak JA. 1979. Comparative effectiveness of paraprofessional and professional helpers. *Psychological Bulletin* 86(1):80-92.

Epperson DL, Bushway DJ, Warman RE. 1983. Client self-terminations after one counseling session: Effects of problem recognition, counselor gender, and counselor experience. *Journal of Counseling Psychology* 30(3):307-315.

Evidence Based Medicine Working Group. 1992. Evidence based medicine: A new approach to teaching the practice of medicine. *Journal of the American Medical Association* 268(17):2420-2425.

Foa EB, Rothbaum BO. 1998. *Treating the trauma of rape.* New York: Guilford Press.

Fontana A, Rosenheck R. 1997. Effectiveness and cost of the inpatient treatment of posttraumatic stress disorder: Comparison of three models of treatment. *American Journal of Psychiatry* 154(6):758-765.

Grace M, Kivlighan DM, Kunce J. 1995. The effect of nonverbal skills training on counselor trainee nonverbal sensitivity and responsiveness and on session impact and working alliance ratings. *Journal of Counseling & Development* 73(5):547-552.

Greenberg G, Rosenheck R. 2005. *Department of Veterans Affairs National Mental Health Program Performance Monitoring System: Fiscal year 2004 report.* West Haven, CT: Northeast Program Evaluation Center, VA Connecticut Healthcare System.

Guyatt GH, Meade MO, Jaeschke RZ, Cook DJ, Haynes RB. 2000. Practitioners of evidence based care: Not all clinicians need to appraise evidence from scratch but all need some skills. *British Medical Journal* 320:954-955.

Harkness L, Kador N. 2001. Treatment of PTSD with families and couples. In *Treating psychological trauma and PTSD,* edited by Wilson JP, Friedman MJ, Lindy JD. New York: Guilford Press. Pp. 335-353.

Hill NR, Beamish PM. 2007. Treatment outcomes for obsessive-compulsive disorder: A critical review. *Journal of Counseling and Development* 85(4):504-510.

Hoge CW, McGurk D, Thomas JL, Cox AL, Engel CC, Castro CA. 2008. Mild traumatic brain injury in US soldiers returning from Iraq. *New England Journal of Medicine* 358:453-463.

IOM (Institute of Medicine). 1990. *Medicare: A strategy for quality assurance,* Vol. I. Washington, DC: National Academy Press.

IOM. 2001. *Crossing the quality chasm: A new health system for the 21st century.* Washington, DC: National Academy Press.

IOM. 2006. *Improving the quality of health care for mental and substance-use conditions: Quality chasm series.* Washington, DC: The National Academies Press.

IOM. 2007. *PTSD compensation and military service.* Washington, DC: The National Academies Press.

IOM. 2008. *Treatment of posttraumatic stress disorder: An assessment of the evidence.* Washington, DC: The National Academies Press.

IOM. 2010. *Redesigning continuing education in the health professions.* Washington, DC: The National Academies Press.

Jacobs S, Prigerson H. 2000. Psychotherapy of traumatic grief: A review of evidence for psychotherapeutic treatments. *Death Studies* 24(6):479-495.

Kim DM, Wampold BE, Bolt DM. 2006. Therapist effects in psychotherapy: A random-effects model of the National Institutes of Mental Health Treatment of Depression Collaborative Research Program data. *Psychotherapy Research* 16(2):161-172.

Kingsley G. 2007. Contemporary group treatment of combat-related posttraumatic stress disorder. *Journal of the Academy of Psychoanalysis and Dynamic Psychiatry 35*(1):51-70.

Kivlighan DM, Kivlighan DM. 2009. Training related changes in the ways that group trainees structure their knowledge of group counseling leader interventions. *Group Dynamics: Theory, Research, and Practice* 13(3):190-204.

Lambert MJ, Harmon C, Slade K, Whipple JL, Hawkins EJ. 2005. Providing feedback to psychotherapists on their patients' progress: Clinical results and practice suggestions. *Journal of Clinical Psychology* 61(2):165-174.

Lehman AF, Kreyenbuhl J, Buchanan RW, Dickerson FB, Dixon LB, Goldberg R, Green-Paden LD, Tenhula WN, Boerescu D, Tek C, Sandson N, Steinwachs DM. 2004. The Schizophrenia Patient Outcomes Research Team (PORT): Updated treatment recommendations 2003. *Schizophrenia Bulletin* 30(2):193-217.

Leichsenring F, Rabung S, Leibing E. 2004. The efficacy of short-term psychodynamic psychotherapy in specific psychiatric disorders: A meta-analysis. *Archives of General Psychiatry* 61(12):1208-1216.

Luborsky L, McLellan AT, Diguer L, Woody G, Seligman DA. 1997. The psychotherapist matters: Comparison of outcomes across twenty-two therapists and seven patient samples. *Clinical Psychology: Science and Practice* 4(1):53-65.

Lumetra. 2008. *External review of the DOD medical quality improvement program.* http://www.tricare.mil/planning/congress/downloads/Review%20of%20DoD%20Medical%20Quality%20Improvement%20Program.pdf. (Accessed October 9, 2009).

Mallinckrodt B, Nelson ML. 1991. Counselor training level and the formation of the psychotherapeutic working alliance. *Journal of Counseling Psychology* 38(2):133-138.

Mayfield WA, Kardash CM, Kivlighan DM. 1999. Differences in experienced and novice counselors' knowledge structures about clients: Implications for case conceptualization. *Journal of Counseling Psychology* 46(4):504-514.

McPherson RH, Pisecco S, Elman NS, Crosbie-Burnett M, Sayger TV. 2000. Counseling psychology's ambivalent relationship with master's-level training. *The Counseling Psychologist* 28(5):687-700.

Meredith LS, Tanielian T, Greenberg MD, Suarez A, Eiseman E. 2005. *Expanding access to mental health counselors: Evaluation of the TRICARE demonstration.* Santa Monica, CA: RAND Corporation.

Monson CM, Fredman SJ, Adair KC. 2008. Cognitive-behavioral conjoint therapy for posttraumatic stress disorder: Application to Operation Enduring and Operation Iraqi Freedom veterans. *Journal of Clinical Psychology* 64(8):958-971.

Mullen E, Bellamy J, Bledsoe S, Francois, J. 2007. Teaching evidence-based practice. *Research on Social Work Practice* 17(5):569-573.

Najavits LM. 2007. Seeking Safety: An evidence-based model for substance abuse and trauma/PTSD. In *Therapist's guide to evidence based relapse prevention: Practical resources for the mental health professional,* edited by Wiktkiewitz KA, Marlatt GA. San Diego: Elsevier. Pp. 141-167.

National Guideline Clearinghouse. 2009. *Criteria for inclusion of clinical practice guidelines in NGC.* http://www.guideline.gov/about/inclusion.aspx. (Accessed October 20, 2009).

Nietzel MT, Fisher SG. 1981. Effectiveness of professional and paraprofessional helpers: A comment on Durlak. *Psychological Bulletin* 89(3):555-565.

NIMH (National Institute of Mental Health). 2009a. *Anxiety disorders.* http://www.nimh.nih.gov/health/publications/anxiety-disorders/complete-index.shtml#pub8. (Accessed September 29, 2009).

NIMH. 2009b. *Bipolar disorder.* http://www.nimh.nih.gov/health/publications/bipolar-disorder/complete-index.shtml. (Accessed September 29, 2009).

NIMH. 2009c. *Post-traumatic stress disorder (PTSD).* http://www.nimh.nih.gov/health/publications/post-traumatic-stress-disorder-ptsd/complete-index.shtml. (Accessed September 29, 2009).

NIMH. 2009d. *Schizophrenia.* http://www.nimh.nih.gov/health/publications/schizophrenia/complete-index.shtml. (Accessed September 29, 2009).

President's New Freedom Commission on Mental Health. 2002. *Achieving the promise: Transforming mental health care in America.* http://www.mentalhealthcommission.gov/reports/FinalReport/downloads/FinalReport.pdf. (Accessed November 13, 2009).

Project MATCH Research Group. 1998. Therapist effects in three treatments for alcohol problems. *Psychotherapy Research* 8(4):455-474.

Resick PS, Schnicke MK. 2002. *Cognitive processing therapy for rape victims: A treatment manual.* Newbury Park, CA: Sage.

Rosenheck R, Fontana A. 2001. Impact of efforts to reduce inpatient costs on clinical effectiveness: Treatment of posttraumatic stress disorder in the Department of Veterans Affairs. *Medical Care* 39(2):168-180.

Ruzek JI, Curran E, Friedman MJ, Gusman FD, Southwick SM, Swales P, Walser RD, Watson PJ, Whealin J. 2004. Treatment of the returning Iraq war veteran. In *Iraq War clinician guide.* White River Station, VT: Department of Veterans Affairs, National

Center for PTSD. http://www.ptsd.va.gov/professional/manuals/manual-pdf/iwcg/iraq_clinician_guide_ch_4.pdf. (Accessed October 23, 2009).

Sackett DL, Rosenberg WM, Muir Gray JA, Haynes RB, Richardson WS. 1996. Evidence based medicine: What it is and isn't. *British Medical Journal* 312:71-72.

Seligman ME. 1995. The effectiveness of psychotherapy: The *Consumer Reports* study. *American Psychologist* 50(12):965-974.

Slade M, McCrone P, Kuipers E, Leese M, Cahill S, Parabiaghi A, Priebe S, Thornicroft G. 2006. Use of standardised outcome measures in adult mental health services: Randomized controlled trial. *British Journal of Psychiatry* 189(4):330-336.

Smith ML, Glass GV. 1977. Meta-analysis of psychotherapy outcome studies. *American Psychologist* 32(9):752-760.

Snyder DK, Castellani AM, Whisman MA. 2006. Current status and future directions in couple therapy. *Annual Review of Psychology* 57(1):317-344.

Spengler PM, White MJ, Ægisdóttir S, Maugherman AS, Anderson LA, Cook RS, Nichols CN, Lampropoulos GK, Walker BS, Cohen GR, Rush JD. 2009. The meta-analysis of clinical judgment project: Effects of experience on judgment accuracy. *The Counseling Psychologist* 37(3):350-399.

Stein DM, Lambert MJ. 1995. Graduate training in psychotherapy: Are therapy outcomes enhanced? *Journal of Consulting and Clinical Psychology* 63(2):182-196.

Summers RF, Barber JP. 2003. Therapeutic alliance as a measurable psychotherapy skill. *Academic Psychiatry* 27(3):160-165.

Surgeon General, Multinational Force-Iraq and the Office of the Surgeon General United States Army Medical Command. 2006. *Mental health advisory team (MHAT) IV: Operation Iraqi Freedom 05-07, Final report.* http://www.house.gov/delahunt/ptsd.pdf. (Accessed October 23, 2009).

TRICARE. 2009. *Evaluation of the TRICARE Program. Fiscal year 2009 report to Congress.* http://www.tricare.mil/Transparency/downloads/TRICARE09_4-7-09_full%20size.pdf. (Accessed October 9, 2009).

Trivedi M, Rush AJ, Wisniewski SR, Nierenberg AA, Warden D, Ritz L, Norquist G, Howland RH, Lebowitz B, McGrath PJ, Shores-Wilson K, Biggs MM, Balasubramani GK, Fava M. 2006. Evaluation of outcomes with citalopram for depression using measurement-based care in STAR*D: Implications for clinical practice. *American Journal of Psychiatry* 163(1):28-40.

VA/DOD (Department of Veterans Affairs/Department of Defense). 2004. *VA/DOD clinical practice guideline for management of post-traumatic stress,* version 1.0. Washington, DC: VA/DOD.

VA/DOD. 2009a. *VA/DOD clinical practice guideline for management of concussion/mild traumatic brain injury.* Washington, DC: VA/DOD.

VA/DOD. 2009b. *VA/DOD clinical practice guideline for management of major depressive disorder (MDD),* version 2.0. Washington, DC: VA/DOD.

VA/DOD. 2009c. *VA/DOD clinical practice guideline for management of substance use disorders (SUD),* version 2.0. Washington, DC: VA/DOD.

Wagner EH, Austin BT, Von Korff M. 1996. Organizing care for patients with chronic illness. *The Milbank Quarterly* 74(4):511-544.

Wampold BE. 2001. *The great psychotherapy debate: Models, methods and findings.* Mahwah, NJ: Lawrence Erlbaum Associates.

Wampold BE, Brown GS. 2005. Estimating variability in outcomes attributable to therapists: A naturalistic study of outcomes in managed care. *Journal of Consulting and Clinical Psychology* 73(5):914-923.

Weiden P, Havens L. 1994. Psychotherapeutic management techniques in the treatment of outpatients with schizophrenia. *Hospital Community Psychiatry* 45(6):549-555.

Weissman MM, Verdeli H, Gameroff MJ, Bledsoe SE, Betts K, Mufson L, Fitterling H, Wickramaratne P. 2006. National survey of psychotherapy training in psychiatry, psychology, and social work. *Archives of General Psychiatry* 63(8):925-934.

# 6

# Findings, Conclusions, and Recommendations

This chapter builds on the foundation laid in Chapters 1–5 to draw general conclusions and recommendations as requested in the statement of task.

## OVERVIEW OF THE COMMITTEE'S WORK AND FINDINGS

The committee's statement of task called for a series of assessments and reviews of the preparation of counselors for professional practice; the institutions that educate them; the licensure, clinical experience, certification, and regulatory and legal requirements applied to them; and their practice in government and other settings.

The statement of task also asked for conclusions and recommendations regarding the independent practice of licensed mental health counselors under the TRICARE program, including recommendations for modifications of TRICARE policy on and limitations of independent practice. It asked the committee to pay particular attention to the preparedness of licensed mental health counselors to diagnose, treat, and appropriately refer persons with a set of illnesses and disorders that service members could be at special risk for.

A 2006 report to Congress by the Department of Defense (DOD) on the use of counselors in the Military Health System (MHS) yields insight on those requests (DOD, 2006). It notes that there is substantial variability among the states in training programs and requirements for licensure as a counselor, that only some educational programs are accredited by the Council for Accreditation of Counseling and Related Educational Programs (CACREP), that in most states licensure requires only minimal coursework in diagnosis of and treatment for mental disorders and no specific clinical experience with people who have mental disorders, and that in some states a license can be obtained with a postgraduate degree in a field other than counseling. The report asserts that physician supervision ensures quality of care for TRICARE beneficiaries.

The committee found that education, accreditation, licensure, certification, and clinical-experience requirements for mental health professionals are components of a quality-management system. However, they have little specificity with regard to knowledge of and experience with particular health problems or evidence-based practices. That generally limits the confidence that can be placed in the preparation of *any* mental health professionals to diagnose and treat disorders that may be found in the TRICARE beneficiary population. Indeed, research regarding the quality of care for mental or substance-use conditions indicates that there are widespread deficiencies in the training of providers and in the infrastructure that supports their practice (IOM, 2006). A 2007 assessment of mental health–care provision in the MHS found the same deficiencies (DOD Task Force on Mental Health, 2007).

Reviews of government programs and government-contracted and private insurers found no consistent pattern in their policies regarding the independent practice of counselors. The policies are by and large driven by federal, state, and tribal laws and regulations and by institutional practice. A historical review of the regulations prescribed by DOD regarding the recognition of mental health providers as independent practitioners indicates that policy is driven primarily by congressional mandate.

Despite an extensive search, the committee identified no literature bearing directly on the comparative quality and effectiveness of care provided by licensed mental health counselors. A review of research related to more general characteristics of mental health practitioners and the care that they deliver found that assertions of differential effectiveness among types of mental health providers are generally not based on empirical evidence. A 2009 meta-analysis (Spengler et al., 2009) concluded that "there are no comprehensive quantitative analyses on . . .

whether any form of educational experience is linked to clinical judgment accuracy."

In summary, the committee did not identify any evidence that distinguishes mental health counselors from other classes of practitioners in ability to serve in an independent professional capacity or to provide high-quality care consistent with education, licensure, and clinical experience. Its research instead points to the need for a comprehensive quality-management system that facilitates the proper diagnosis of and treatment for disorders in the TRICARE beneficiary population by all mental health practitioners.

## RECOMMENDATIONS

The committee was tasked to offer:

> conclusions and recommendations for permitting licensed mental health counselors to practice independently under the TRICARE program, including recommendation regarding modifications of current policy for the TRICARE program with respect to allowing licensed mental health counselors to practice independently in the TRICARE program, paying particular attention to the preparedness of licensed mental health counselors to diagnose, treat and appropriately refer persons with disorders of particular importance to TRICARE beneficiaries.

In light of the information that it gathered and reviewed, it recommends that TRICARE replace its current quality management system for oversight of the practice of counselors through physician referral and supervision[1] with a mental health quality monitoring and management system that incorporates the following two primary elements:

**[1] Independent practice of mental health counselors in TRICARE in the circumstances in which their education, licensure, and clinical experience have helped to prepare them to diagnose and, where appropriate, treat conditions in the beneficiary population.** Those circumstances comprise

---

[1]Current TRICARE policies regarding the practice of counselors are detailed in Chapter 1.

- A master's or higher-level degree in counseling from a program in mental health counseling or clinical mental health counseling that is accredited by CACREP.
- A state license in mental health counseling at the "clinical" or the higher or highest level available in states that have tiered licensing schemes.
- Passage of the National Clinical Mental Health Counseling Examination (NCMHCE).
- A well-defined scope of practice for practitioners.

The scope of practice should be based on a systematic assessment of the professional and cultural competencies necessary to address the mental and behavioral health needs of the TRICARE beneficiary population and should include the types of patients that can be seen, the settings in which they can be seen, and the interventions and populations (including pediatric, adolescent, and geriatric) that the practitioner has demonstrated competency in.

TRICARE currently requires certified clinical social workers to hold "a master's degree in social work from a graduate school of social work accredited by the Council on Social Work Education" in order to practice independently (32 CFR § 199.6, documented in Appendix D). The committee believes that a parallel requirement for counselors is appropriate.[2] CACREP accreditation in clinical mental health counseling requires programs to provide evidence that student learning has occurred in a number of knowledge, skills, and practice categories that are desirable for an independent practitioner in TRICARE, including (CACREP, 2009)

- Etiology, the diagnostic process and nomenclature, treatment, referral, and prevention of mental and emotional disorders.
- Principles of the diagnostic process, including differential diagnosis, and the use of current diagnostic tools, such as the current edition of the *Diagnostic and Statistical Manual of Mental Disorders.*
- Accurate multi-axial diagnosis of disorders.

[2]This may make CACREP eligible to apply for recognition by the US Department of Education through the National Advisory Committee on Institutional Quality and Integrity, a federal entity that sets and enforces standards for accrediting agencies and associations.

- [Understanding of] basic classifications, indications, and contra-indications of commonly prescribed psychopharmacological medications so that appropriate referrals can be made for medication evaluations and so that the side effects of such medications can be identified.
- Evidence-based treatments and basic strategies for evaluating counseling outcomes in clinical mental health counseling.
- [Development of] measurable outcomes for clinical mental health counseling programs, interventions, and treatments.
- [Critical evaluation of] research relevant to the practice of clinical mental health counseling.

A student must also demonstrate "the ability to recognize his or her own limitations as a clinical mental health counselor and to seek supervision or refer clients when appropriate."

As the committee's research has documented, there is considerable variability in the examination requirements and numbers of hours of supervised clinical experience needed for state licensure as a mental health counselor. Federal regulation and TRICARE policy already require counselors to have "two years of post-masters experience which includes 3000 hours of clinical work and 100 hours of face-to-face supervision" (32 CFR § 199.6) for them to practice in the system, and the committee recommends that this requirement be retained. A requirement for licensure at the higher or the highest level offered by a state would help to ensure that practitioners have the training and experience needed to serve in an independent capacity. Some states—such as Illinois, Kansas, and Nebraska—already follow that strategy, granting authority for independent practice only to persons who hold their highest-level license.

The NCMHCE is designed specifically for counselors who work in mental health, in contrast with the National Counselor Examination (NCE), which is a generic counseling examination. It tests the ability to provide services in a clinical capacity, including performing a differential diagnosis according to the *Diagnostic and Statistical Manual of Mental Disorders, Fourth Edition,* and the *International Classification of Diseases, Ninth Revision, Clinical Modification.* The NCMHCE's clinical simulations span the range of ages—adolescents, young adults, middle-aged adults, and older adults—and address the primary and secondary clinical features seen in the TRICARE population. The committee concludes that although the NCMHCE has limitations,[3] it is a more relevant test than the NCE of the ability of counselors to serve as independent providers of mental health care. State licensure boards apparently also have that view, with some using the NCMHCE as the examination applied to the higher or highest or clinical level of licensure.

Scopes of practice—which are called scopes of care in some military health publications—are routinely used in clinical settings to define the circumstances under which practitioners provide services and the services for which they have demonstrated expertise. A well-defined scope of practice is an essential component of clinical privileging, which, as the committee indicates below, is part of the comprehensive quality-management system that TRICARE should maintain for all health professionals.

The committee believes that the requirements listed above, in concert with a comprehensive quality-management system, address the concerns expressed by DOD regarding the independent practice of mental health counselors and would help to ensure that TRICARE beneficiaries who seek counselors' services would receive high-quality care, including, as appropriate, referral to other professionals.

The committee believes that it is important to maintain continuity of care for TRICARE beneficiaries who are receiving services from counselors under the current system. It therefore recommends that TRICARE institute a strategy that allows for the continuing service of practitioners who did not graduate from CACREP-accredited programs,[4] have not attained "clinical" or similar licensure, or have not successfully completed the NCMHCE. TRICARE may, for example, wish to conduct supervision of such professionals by using a model patterned after Army Regulation 40–68, Sections 7–6c and d (Appendix E), which provides for successively greater levels of independent practice as experience and demonstrated competence increase.

---

[3]The NCMHCE is not currently being reviewed by a third-party accrediting body for fairness, validity and reliability. The credibility of the examination would be enhanced if it were to obtain recognition through such a body.

[4]Some current counselors may have graduated from programs accredited by the Council on Rehabilitation Education, later gained clinical experience and earned licensure in mental health counseling, and be practicing as counselors. The committee does not intend to exclude such persons from practicing in the TRICARE system.

**[2] A comprehensive quality-management system for all mental health professionals.** This system should include

- Well-defined scopes of practice and clinical privileging of all mental health–care providers in the direct- and purchased-care systems that are consistent with professional education, training, and experience, where these scopes are not already present.
- Promotion of evidence-based practices for treatment of conditions and monitoring of results.
- Focused training in the particular mental and related general medical conditions that are present in the TRICARE beneficiary population and in military cultural competence.
- A systematic process for continued professional education and training to ensure continuing improvement in the clinical evidence base and accommodation of the changing needs of the TRICARE population.
- Development and application of quality measures to assess the performance of providers.
- Systematic monitoring of the process and outcomes of care at all levels of the health-care system and application of effective quality-improvement strategies.

Chapter 5, which summarizes the conclusions of previous Institute of Medicine studies of the determinants of high-quality health care (IOM, 2001, 2006), documents the importance of those steps and provides the foundation of the committee's recommendation here.

The committee notes that the recommendations regarding evidence-based practices, training and education, quality measures, and monitoring echo the observations offered by the mental health task force convened by DOD (DOD Task Force on Mental Health, 2007). DOD publications and public pronouncements (Casscells, 2008; DOD, 2008) indicate that the MHS is already pursuing these recommendations as part of its efforts to implement best practices in quality management. For example, the DOD Center for Deployment Psychology (CDP) is currently offering courses on military cultural competence to TRICARE personnel and other MHS practitioners (CDP, 2009). In April 2010, CDP will initiate a military and veteran behavioral health post-master's certificate program that will "teach best clinical practices to mental health professionals who are addressing the behavioral health needs of military personnel, veterans and their families" and include training in military culture, combat trauma, suicide risk, and blast-related traumatic brain injury (CDP, 2010). The committee believes that the framework necessary to support the independent practice of counselors under the circumstances delineated above is thus already being put into place, that TRICARE should be able to implement the recommended policy changes in a timely manner, and that it should do so because of the critical mental health needs in its beneficiary population. As a step toward achieving the comprehensive system recommended here, the TRICARE Management Activity should consider requiring that organizations demonstrate that they have mechanisms in place to promote the delivery of evidence-based care, to apply quality measures to assess the performance of providers, to monitor outcomes, and to implement improvement strategies as a condition of their provider contracts.

The committee observes that the barriers to establishing a robust quality infrastructure for mental health care are common to all providers and suggests that TRICARE may benefit by working with other government organizations—such as the Department of Veterans Affairs and the Department of Health and Human Services' Agency for Healthcare Research and Quality, the Centers for Medicare & Medicaid Services, the National Institutes of Health, and the Substance Abuse and Mental Health Services Administration—to conduct or support research to overcome the barriers.

## REFERENCES

CACREP (Council on Accreditation of Counseling and Related Educational Programs). 2009. *CACREP accreditation manual: 2009 standards.* Alexandria, VA: CACREP.

Casscells SW. 2008. *Statement on mental health by The Honorable S. Ward Casscells, MD, Assistant Secretary of Defense for Health Affairs, before the Subcommittee on Military Personnel of the Armed Services Committee, US House of Representatives,* March 14. http://www.dod.mil/dodgc/olc/docs/testCasscells080314.pdf. (Accessed October 9, 2009).

CDP (Center for Deployment Psychology, DOD). 2009. *Welcome to the Center for Deployment Psychology.* http://www.deploymentpsych.org/. (Accessed December 22, 2009).

CDP. 2010. *Military and veteran behavioral health post-master's certificate program.* http://postgraduatecenter.org/MVBH%20Certificate.html. (Accessed January 15, 2010).

DOD (Department of Defense). 2006. *Aspects of the use of licensed professional counselors in the military health system. Report to Congress.* Transmittal letter, August 28. http://www.tricare.mil/planning/congress/downloads/2006/new/Licensed-Mental.pdf. (Accessed October 20, 2009).

DOD. 2008. *The Military Health System strategic plan. A roadmap for medical transformation.* http://www.health.mil/StrategicPlan/2008%20Strat%20Plan%20Final%20-lowres.pdf. (Accessed October 27, 2009.

DOD Task Force on Mental Health. 2007. *An achievable vision: Report of the Department of Defense Task Force on Mental Health.* Falls Church, VA: Defense Health Board. http://www.health.mil/dhb/mhtf/MHTF-Report-Final.pdf. (Accessed October 27, 2009).

IOM (Institute of Medicine). 2001. *Crossing the quality chasm: A new health system for the 21st century.* Washington, DC: National Academy Press.

IOM. 2006. *Improving the quality of health care for mental and substance-use conditions: Quality chasm series.* Washington, DC: The National Academies Press.

Spengler PM, White MJ, Ægisdóttir S, Maugherman AS, Anderson LA, Cook RS, Nichols CN, Lampropoulos GK, Walker BS, Cohen GR, Rush JD. 2009. The meta-analysis of clinical judgment project: Effects of experience on judgment accuracy. *The Counseling Psychologist* 37(3):350-399.

# Appendixes

# Appendix A

# Public Meeting Agendas

## WORKSHOP 1
## April 9, 2009
## Keck Center of the National Academies
## 500 Fifth Street, NW, Washington, DC

**Session I—Issues to be considered in the study**

**10:00 a.m.–10:05 a.m.**
***Welcome to the National Academies and the Institute of Medicine***

Frederick Erdtmann, M.D., M.P.H.
Director, Board on the Health of Select Populations, Institute of Medicine, National Academy of Sciences

**10:05 a.m.–10:15 a.m.**
***Conduct of the workshop and introduction of the Committee***

George J. Isham, M.D.
Committee Chair

**10:15 a.m.–11:15 a.m.**
***Charge to the workshop speakers; background on the delivery of TRICARE mental health services***

LT Richard Schobitz, Ph.D. (USPHS)
Deputy Director, Behavior Medicine Division, Office of the Chief Medical Officer, TRICARE Management Authority, Department of Defense

**11:15 a.m.–12:15 p.m.**
***Results of the RAND report "Expanding Access to Mental Health Counselors"***

Lisa S. Meredith, Ph.D.
Senior Behavioral Scientist, RAND Corporation; Research Scientist, Center for the Study of Healthcare Provider Behavior, VA Medical Center

Terri Tanielian, M.A.
Co-Director, RAND Center for Military Health Policy Research, Arroyo Center; Senior Social Research Analyst

**1:15 p.m.–2:15 p.m.**
***State licensure laws and the mental health professions***

David Hartley, Ph.D.
Research Professor, Institute for Health Policy and Director, Maine Rural Health Research Center, Muskie School of Public Service, University of Southern Maine

**Session II—Remarks from interested organizations**

**2:30 p.m.–3:00 p.m.**
***Remarks from the Council for Accreditation of Counseling and Related Educational Programs***

Carol L. Bobby, Ph.D., LPC, NCC
Executive Director

**3:00 p.m.–3:30 p.m.**
***Remarks from the National Board for Certified Counselors***

Thomas Clawson, Ph.D.
President and Chief Executive Officer

**3:30 p.m.–4:00 p.m.**
***Remarks from the American Counseling Association***

David Kaplan, Ph.D.
Chief Professional Officer

**4:00 p.m.–5:00 p.m.**
***Roundtable discussion—day's speakers***

George J. Isham, M.D., Moderator

**5:00 p.m.**
***Workshop adjourns***

## WORKSHOP 2
## July 7, 2009
## Keck Center of the National Academies
## 500 Fifth Street, NW, Washington, DC

**12:30 p.m.–12:45 p.m.**
***Opening remarks***

George J. Isham, M.D.
Committee Chair and Workshop Moderator

**12:45 p.m.–1:45 p.m.**
***Counselors in the federal government and private sectors***

Richard A. McCormick, Ph.D.
Senior Scholar, Center for Health Care Research and Policy, Case Western Reserve University (formerly Chief, Psychology Service, Cleveland VA Medical Center, and Member, Secretary of Veterans Affairs Special Mental Health Advisory Task Force)

Doug Nemecek, M.D., M.B.A.
National Medical Director, Health Solutions, CIGNA

**2:00 p.m.–3:30 p.m.**
***Counselors in the TRICARE system***

John C. Bradley, M.D. (COL, MC, USA)
Chair, Integrated Department of Psychiatry and Behavioral Health, Walter Reed Army Medical Center and National Naval Medical Center; Vice Chair, Department of Psychiatry, Uniformed Services University, Bethesda, MD; Psychiatry Consultant to the Commander, North Atlantic Regional Medical Command

Andrew L. Findley, M.D. (CAPT, MC, USN)
Chief Operating Officer/Medical Director, TRICARE Regional Office—North

Marie L. Mentor, R.N., M.S.N.
Mental Health Nurse Consultant, TRICARE Region North, Clinical Operations

Ian A. Shaffer, M.D., M.M.M.
Chief Medical Officer, MHN—A Health Net Company

**3:30 p.m.–4:00 p.m.**
***Practitioner perspective***

R. Scott Walton, Ph.D., CCMHC, NCC, LMHC, LPC, LRC
Walton-Brueske Counseling Group, PA

**4:00 p.m.–5:00 p.m.**
***Roundtable discussion—committee, speakers, and observers***

George J. Isham, M.D., Moderator

**5:00 p.m.**
***Workshop adjourns***

# Appendix B

# Additional Demographic Information on the TRICARE Beneficiary Population

As noted in Chapter 2, the TRICARE beneficiary population is a far larger and more diverse population than the active-duty personnel who might come to mind first when one is considering the mental health risks and needs of a military population. This appendix presents details on the demographic and socioeconomic characteristics of the general military population, including military families, with information on Operation Iraqi Freedom (OIF) and Operation Enduring Freedom (OEF) warfighters. These data are intended to provide more in-depth background on both the similarities and the differences between the TRICARE population and other managed–health-care populations.

## DEMOGRAPHIC AND SOCIOECONOMIC INFORMATION ON THE GENERAL MILITARY POPULATION

In general, a high-school diploma or general equivalency diploma (GED) is required for enlistment in the military, and 98.4% and 93.7% of new active-duty enlistees and new Reserve enlistees, respectively, in FY 2007 had at least a high-school diploma or the equivalent. In contrast, 81.2% of the 18- to 24-year-old civilian population have met those educational standards. Of the enlisted force as a whole (Table B.1), 98.4% of active-duty enlisted service members have at least a high-school diploma or GED compared with 93.8% in the reserve components and 84.5% of the civilian population over 25 years old (DOD, 2007).

The vast majority of commissioned and warrant officers—87.3% on active duty and 85.6% in the reserve components—hold at least a college degree (Table B.1). In general, a college degree is required for appointment as a commissioned, but not warrant, officer. Among all enlisted members, 4.4% on active duty and 7.4% in the reserve components are at least college graduates. In the combined officer corps and enlisted corps, 17.8% of the active-duty force and 19.1% of the reserve force have at least a bachelor's degree. In comparison, 27.5% of the civilian population over 25 years old have at least graduated from college (DOD, 2007).

In both the active and reserve components, minority groups (self-reported as African American or black, Hispanic, Asian, American Indian, Alaska Native, Native Hawaiian or other Pacific islander, multiracial, or other or unknown) make up greater proportions of the enlisted ranks than of the officer corps. Put another way, of all minority-group members of the reserve components, 10.4% are officers and 89.6% enlisted; similarly, of active-duty minority-group members, 10.7% are officers and 89.3% enlisted. In both cases, the proportion of minority-group members who are officers—16.2% on active duty and 14.9% in the reserve components—is lower than the overall proportion who are officers. Of women, 17.1% on active duty are officers, and 15.2% in the reserve components are officers (DOD, 2007). Breakdowns of the military population by race and ethnicity are shown in Table B.2.

**TABLE B.1** Minimum Educational Levels of Officers and Enlisted Members of the Armed Forces

| | At Least High School (%) | At Least College (%) |
|---|---|---|
| Total active duty | 98.6[a] | 17.8 |
| Enlisted | 98.4 | 4.4 |
| Officer | 99.9 | 87.3 |
| Total reserve components | 94.7[a] | 19.1 |
| Enlisted | 93.8 | 7.4 |
| Officer | 99.9 | 85.6 |
| Civilians over 25 years old | 84.5 | 27.5 |

[a]Information calculated from data in DOD demographics report.
SOURCE: DOD (2007).

**TABLE B.2** Race or Ethnicity of Service Members and the General Population[a]

| | Active Duty (%) | Reserve or National Guard (%) | General Population (%) |
|---|---|---|---|
| White | 64.1 | 70.1 | 66.01 |
| Black | 16.8 | 14.7 | 12.28 |
| Hispanic | 10.4 | 8.9 | 15.09 |
| Asian | 3.4 | 2.4 | 4.33 |
| American Indian or Alaska Native | 1.4 | 0.8 | 0.76 |
| Native Hawaiian or Pacific Islander | 0.5 | 0.5 | 0.14 |
| Multiracial | 0.9 | 0.5 | 1.39 |
| Unknown or other | 2.5 | 2.1 | — |

[a]For all data except Hispanic, percentages are for those who do not also identify as Hispanic.
SOURCES: DOD (2007); US Census Bureau (2008).

In the overall population of people 17–64 years old, 42.6% are single (including divorced and widowed) (US Census Bureau, 2009). In comparison, 44.8% of active-duty service members and 51% of Reserves are single. Of active-duty service members, 43.1% have dependent children, defined as dependents under 23 years old who are enrolled as full-time students. As might be expected, older service members are more likely to have children than younger members. However, officers in the general or admiral ranks are less likely than officers ranking between major or lieutenant commander and colonel or captain to have dependent children. That is probably because the children of generals and admirals have already passed the age of 23 years. The same patterns are found in the reserve components, although the overall proportion of members who have children is 41.9%. In both active-duty and reserve-component families with children, the average number of children is 2. However, the age distribution of children differs between active and reserve components, as shown in Table B.3 (DOD, 2007). In the civilian population, the average number of children in families with children is 1.86 (US Census Bureau, 2008).

The largest proportion, 25.51%, of new active-duty enlistees come from communities that have median incomes of $42,040–51,127. Communities that have median incomes of $33,268–65,031 provide

**TABLE B.3** Age Distribution of Children in Active-Duty and Reserve-Component Families

| Age | Active Duty (%) | Reserve or National Guard (%) |
|---|---|---|
| 0–5 years | 41.0 | 24.7 |
| 6–14 years | 31.4 | 46.2 |
| 15–18 years | 23.8 | 17.8 |
| 19–22 years | 3.8 | 11.3 |

SOURCE: DOD (2007).

70.09% of new active-duty enlistees (DOD Task Force on Mental Health, 2007). It is difficult to compare military pay with civilian pay directly because military compensation includes salary, tax breaks, housing benefits, and health care. However, for illustrative purposes, an Army sergeant (E-5) with 4 years of service who is married and has children could earn about $47,000, including benefits, per year. A first lieutenant (O-2) in the same situation could earn about $68,000 per year (US Army, 2008). In active-duty families, 42% of officers' spouses are out of the workforce (neither employed nor seeking employment) compared with 31% of enlisted members' spouses (DOD, 2007).

In summary, the active-duty military population is more likely to have graduated from high school but less likely to have graduated from college than the civilian population (Table B.1). Active-duty service members are about as likely to be single as the general population, whereas reservists are more likely to be single. Compensation in the military is competitive with civilian salaries. In both active-duty and Reserve families with children, the average number of children is 2, a little higher than in the general population, and more young children (0–5 years old) are found in active-duty families than in Reserve families (Table B.3).

## DEMOGRAPHICS OF THE OPERATION IRAQI FREEDOM AND OPERATION ENDURING FREEDOM POPULATIONS

As of October 2007, more than 1.6 million US service members had been deployed to Iraq and Afghanistan (Tanielian and Jaycox, 2008). Among the OIF and OEF service members, there has been a marked increase of women among the ranks: 15% on active duty, 24% in the

Army Reserves, and 13% in the National Guard (DOD, 2007). The increase in cultural and racial diversity indicates a need to be cognizant of "culturally responsive" clinical practice.

Demographic shifts in recent war zones have resulted in a stronger presence of women serving in combat zones, a higher rate of married reservists (49%), an increase in dual-career military couples, and higher proportions of women in the National Guard and the Reserves. More than half (57%) of active-duty service members have family responsibilities (a partner, children, or other dependents). Among Reserve and National Guard families, 49% are married, and 42% have children (DOD, 2007).

As of January 2, 2010, 5,297 troops had been killed in the OIF and OEF conflicts, 4,361 in the OIF theater and 936 in the OEF theater (DOD, 2010). Most (73%) of the fallen served in the Army. About half (51%) of those troops were under 25 years old. A total of 36,364 had been wounded in action as the result of hostile activity as of January 2, 2010: 31,616 in the OIF theater and 4,748 in the OEF theater. Over 65% of these injuries were the result of explosive devices. Data on psychological injuries suffered during combat are not available.

In a RAND monograph, Tanielian and Jaycox (2008) estimated that 320,000 service members experienced a probable traumatic brain injury during deployment. However, in their sample of 1,965 previously deployed persons, only 43% had been evaluated by a physician or specialist for possible brain injury. That low rate of access raises questions about barriers to service, about whether stigma influences help seeking, and about whether lack of preparedness among family members and providers prevents them from recognizing symptoms and concerns associated with brain injury. Many of those veterans will be treated in polytrauma centers that involve long-term rehabilitation, so clinicians who work with them and their family members need to understand the complexity of the physical, psychosocial, and mental health issues for everyone involved.

## REFERENCES

DOD (Department of Defense). 2007. *Demographics 2007: Profile of the military community.* http://cs.mhf.dod.mil/content/dav/mhf/QOL-Library/Project%20Documents/MilitaryHOMEFRONT/Reports/2007%20Demographics.pdf. (Accessed July 28, 2009).

DOD. 2010. *Military casualty information.* http://siadapp.dmdc.osd.mil/personnel/CASUALTY/castop.htm. (Accessed January 15, 2010).

DOD Task Force on Mental Health. 2007. *An achievable vision: Report of the Department of Defense Task Force on Mental Health.* Falls Church, VA: Defense Health Board.

Tanielian T, Jaycox LH (Eds.). 2008. *Invisible wounds of war: Psychological and cognitive injuries, their consequences, and services to assist recovery.* Santa Monica, CA: RAND Corporation. http://www.rand.org/pubs/monographs/2008/RAND_MG720.pdf. (Accessed January 15, 2010).

US Census Bureau. 2008. *Annual estimates of the population by sex, race, and Hispanic origin for the United States: April 1, 2000 to July 1, 2007 (nc-est2007-03).* http://www.census.gov/compenia/statab/tables/09s0006.pdf. (Accessed July 31, 2009).

US Census Bureau. 2009. *America's families and living arrangements—Table A1, "Marital status of people 15 years and over, by age, sex, personal earnings, race, and Hispanic origin, 2008.* http://www.census.gov/population/www/socdemo/hh-fam/cps2008.html. (Accessed July 28, 2009).

# Appendix C

# Definition of Terms Used in This Report

Several terms are used in this report to refer to concepts in the field of mental health care and counseling. The committee's working definitions of those terms are listed here.

**Counseling:** An array of noninvasive and nonpharmacologic interventions whose primary focus is on promoting coping and facilitating growth related to life-cycle transitions.

**Credentialing:** The systematic process of screening and evaluating qualifications and other relevant evidence—such as licensure, education, training, and clinical experience—to ensure that specific requirements are met.

**Diagnosis:** Comprehensive and systematic assessment of a person presenting for mental health care to gain an understanding of the person's clinical condition and determine a plan of treatment. Three issues are critical to understanding the nature of this task:

(1) The designation of a specific *Diagnostic and Statistical Manual of Mental Disorders* (*DSM*) or *International Classification of Diseases* (*ICD*) diagnosis is generally considered an essential element of "making a diagnosis." However, making a *DSM* or *ICD* diagnosis is only one element of a comprehensive evaluation. To

formulate an adequate treatment plan, the clinician will invariably require considerable information about the person being evaluated beyond that required for a *DSM* or *ICD* diagnosis. Furthermore, these systems are intended to be used by people who have appropriate clinical training and experience in diagnosis and their criteria are meant to serve as guidelines to be informed by clinical judgment, not to be used as a cookbook.

(2) Unfortunately, the term *mental disorder* implies a distinction from *physical disorder*. This is a reductionistic anachronism of mind–body dualism. A compelling literature documents that there is much "physical" in "mental" and "mental" in "physical."

(3) A diagnostic assessment is not a one-time event that occurs at the initiation of care. Diagnostic assessment is a longitudinal process that requires continuing, systematic data collection and integration of the data into a continually evolving treatment plan.

**Licensure:** A document—a license, certification, or registration—that grants official or legal permission to practice in a state or other jurisdiction.

**Privileging:** The process by which the scope and content of patient-care services are defined for an individual provider. Privileging by a healthcare organization is based on an evaluation of a provider's credentials and performance in delivering services competently, and it authorizes the provider to perform the duties outlined in his or her professional scope of practice.

**Psychotherapy:** An array of noninvasive and nonpharmacologic clinical interventions whose primary focus is on remedying symptoms, behaviors, and affect associated with psychopathologic conditions; fostering emotional growth; and improving functioning. (Note that most insurance plans do not reimburse for "growth" alone, in that it is not considered to be a so-called medical necessity.)

**Quality:** The degree to which health services for individuals and populations increase the likelihood of desired health outcomes and are consistent with current professional knowledge. Quality incorporates six aims: safety, timeliness, effectiveness, efficiency, patient-centeredness, and equitableness. Good-quality services are provided in a culturally sensitive and technically competent manner with good communication and shared decision making. Quality is often thought of as containing three main components: structure, process, and outcomes of care (Donabedian, 1998).

**Scope of Practice:** The range of activities (the ability to perform diagnoses, deliver treatment, or prescribe medications, for example) or procedures that a medical professional is permitted to perform under the law, their license, a regulation, a provider agreement, or other system of conduct. A scope of practice may be defined on the basis of a professional's level of education, training, or experience, or on the basis of an assessment of the professional's demonstrated competencies. It may include a list of circumstances under which the activities or procedures must be performed under some form of supervision.

**Treatment:** An array of procedures and interventions intended to alleviate illness and improve or if possible restore health and improve function in affected people.

## REFERENCE

Donabedian A. 1998. The quality of health care: How can it be assessed? *Journal of the American Medical Association* 260(12):1743-1748.

# Appendix D

# Excerpts from 32 CFR § 199.6: Selected Subsections Regarding the Practice of Authorized Mental Health Providers Under TRICARE

(iii) ***Other allied health professionals***. The services of the following individual professional providers of care are coverable on a fee-for-service basis provided such services are otherwise authorized in this or other sections of this part.

(A) ***Clinical psychologist***. For purposes of CHAMPUS, a clinical psychologist is an individual who is licensed or certified by the state for the independent practice of psychology and:

*(1)* Possesses a doctoral degree in psychology from a regionally accredited university; and

*(2)* Has had 2 years of supervised clinical experience in psychological health services of which at least 1 year is post-doctoral and 1 year (may be the post-doctoral year) is in an organized psychological health service training program; or

*(3)* As an alternative to paragraphs (c)(3)(iii)(A)(*1*) and (*2*) of this section [*that is, as an alternative to the clauses above*] is listed in the National Register of Health Service Providers in Psychology.

. . . .

(F) ***Certified Clinical Social Worker***. A clinical social worker may provide covered services independent of physician referral and supervision, provided the clinical social worker:

*(1)* Is licensed or certified as a clinical social worker by the jurisdiction where practicing; or, if the jurisdiction does not provide for licensure or certification of clinical social workers, is certified by a national professional organization offering certification of clinical social workers; and

*(2)* Has at least a master's degree in social work from a graduate school of social work accredited by the Council on Social Work Education; and

*(3)* Has had a minimum of 2 years or 3,000 hours of post-master's degree supervised clinical social work practice under the supervision of a master's level social worker in an appropriate clinical setting, as determined by the Director, OCHAMPUS, or a designee.

Note: Patients' organic medical problems must receive appropriate concurrent management by a physician.

(G) ***Certified psychiatric nurse specialist.*** A certified psychiatric nurse specialist may provide covered care independent of physician referral and supervision. For purposes of CHAMPUS, a certified psychiatric nurse specialist is an individual who:

*(1)* Is a licensed, registered nurse; and

*(2)* Has at least a master's degree in nursing from a regionally accredited institution with a specialization in psychiatric and mental health nursing; and

*(3)* Has had at least 2 years of post-master's degree practice in the field of psychiatric and mental health nursing, including an average of 8 hours of direct patient contact per week; or

*(4)* Is listed in a CHAMPUS-recognized, professionally sanctioned listing of clinical specialists in psychiatric and mental health nursing.

(iv) ***Extramedical individual providers.*** Extramedical individual providers are those who do counseling or nonmedical therapy and whose training and therapeutic concepts are outside the medical field. The services of extramedical individual professionals are coverable following the CHAMPUS determined allowable charge methodology provided such services are otherwise authorized in this or other sections of the regulation.

(A) ***Certified marriage and family therapists.*** For the purposes of CHAMPUS, a certified marriage and family therapist is an individual who meets the following requirements:

*(1)* Recognized graduate professional education with the minimum of an earned master's degree from a regionally accredited educational institution in an appropriate behavioral science field, mental health discipline; and

*(2)* The following experience:

*(i)* Either 200 hours of approved supervision in the practice of marriage and family counseling, ordinarily to be completed in a 2- to 3-year period, of which at least 100 hours must be in individual supervision. This supervision will occur preferably with more than one supervisor and should include a continuous process of supervision with at least three cases; and

*(ii)* 1,000 hours of clinical experience in the practice of marriage and family counseling under approved supervision, involving at least 50 different cases; or

*(iii)* 150 hours of approved supervision in the practice of psychotherapy, ordinarily to be completed in a 2- to 3-year period, of which at least 50 hours must be individual supervision; plus at least 50 hours of approved individual supervision in the practice of marriage and family counseling, ordinarily to be completed within a period of not less than 1 nor more than 2 years; and

*(iv)* 750 hours of clinical experience in the practice of psychotherapy under approved supervision involving at least 30 cases; plus at least 250 hours of clinical practice in marriage and family counseling under approved supervision, involving at least 20 cases; and

*(3)* Is licensed or certified to practice as a marriage and family therapist by the jurisdiction where practicing (see paragraph (c)(3)(iv)(D) of this section for more specific information regarding licensure); and

*(4)* Agrees that a patients' [*sic*] organic medical problems must receive appropriate concurrent management by a physician.

. . .

(B) ***Pastoral counselors***. For the purposes of CHAMPUS, a pastoral counselor is an individual who meets the following requirements:

- *(1)* Recognized graduate professional education with the minimum of an earned master's degree from a regionally accredited educational institution in an appropriate behavioral science field, mental health discipline; and
- *(2)* The following experience:
  - *(i)* Either 200 hours of approved supervision in the practice of pastoral counseling, ordinarily to be completed in a 2- to 3-year period, of which at least 100 hours must be in individual supervision. This supervision will occur preferably with more than one supervisor and should include a continuous process of supervision with at least three cases; and
  - *(ii)* 1,000 hours of clinical experience in the practice of pastoral counseling under approved supervision, involving at least 50 different cases; or
  - *(iii)* 150 hours of approved supervision in the practice of psychotherapy, ordinarily to be completed in a 2- to 3-year period, of which at least 50 hours must be individual supervision; plus at least 50 hours of approved individual supervision in the practice of pastoral counseling, ordinarily to be completed within a period of not less than 1 nor more than 2 years; and
  - *(iv)* 750 hours of clinical experience in the practice of psychotherapy under approved supervision involving at least 30 cases; plus at least 250 hours of clinical practice in pastoral counseling under approved supervision, involving at least 20 cases; and
- *(3)* Is licensed or certified to practice as a pastoral counselor by the jurisdiction where practicing (see paragraph (c)(3)(iv)(D) of this section for more specific information regarding licensure); and
- *(4)* The services of a pastoral counselor meeting the above requirements are coverable following the CHAMPUS determined allowable charge methodology, under the following specified conditions:
  - *(i)* The CHAMPUS beneficiary must be referred for therapy by a physician; and

*(ii)* A physician is providing ongoing oversight and supervision of the therapy being provided; and

*(iii)* The pastoral counselor must certify on each claim for reimbursement that a written communication has been made or will be made to the referring physician of the results of the treatment. Such communication will be made at the end of the treatment, or more frequently, as required by the referring physician (refer to § 199.7).

*(5)* Because of the similarity of the requirements for licensure, certification, experience, and education, a pastoral counselor may elect to be authorized under CHAMPUS as a certified marriage and family therapist, and as such, be subject to all previously defined criteria for the certified marriage and family therapist category, to include acceptance of the CHAMPUS determined allowable charge as payment in full, except for applicable deductibles and cost-shares (i.e., balance billing of a beneficiary above the allowable charge is prohibited; may not bill beneficiary for noncovered care). The pastoral counselor must also agree to enter into the same participation agreement as a certified marriage and family therapist with the Office of CHAMPUS within which the pastoral counselor agrees to all provisions including licensure, national association membership and conditions upon termination, outlined above for certified marriage and family therapist.

Note: No dual status will be recognized by the Office of CHAMPUS. Pastoral counselors must elect to become one of the categories of extra-medical CHAMPUS providers specified above. Once authorized as either a pastoral counselor, or a certified marriage and family therapist, claims review and reimbursement will be in accordance with the criteria established for the elected provider category.

(C) ***Mental health counselor***. For the purposes of CHAMPUS, a mental health counselor is an individual who meets the following requirements:

*(1)* Minimum of a master's degree in mental health counseling or allied mental health field from a regionally accredited institution; and

*(2)* Two years of post-masters experience which includes 3000 hours of clinical work and 100 hours of face-to-face supervision; and

*(3)* Is licensed or certified to practice as a mental health counselor by the jurisdiction where practicing (see paragraph (c)(3)(iv)(D) of this section for more specific information); and

*(4)* May only be reimbursed when:

*(i)* The CHAMPUS beneficiary is referred for therapy by a physician; and

*(ii)* A physician is providing ongoing oversight and supervision of the therapy being provided; and

*(iii)* The mental health counselor certifies on each claim for reimbursement that a written communication has been made or will be made to the referring physician of the results of the treatment. Such communication will be made at the end of the treatment, or more frequently, as required by the referring physician (refer to § 199.7).

(D) The following additional information applies to each of the above categories of extramedical individual providers:

These providers must also be licensed or certified to practice as a certified marriage and family therapist, pastoral counselor or mental health counselor by the jurisdiction where practicing. In jurisdictions that do not provide for licensure or certification, the provider must be certified by or eligible for full clinical membership in the appropriate national professional association that sets standards for the specific profession.

. . . .

(2) ***Conditions of authorization***—

(i) ***Professional license requirement.*** The individual must be currently licensed to render professional health care services in each state in which the individual renders services to CHAMPUS beneficiaries. Such license is required when a specific state provides, but does not require, license for a specific category of individual professional provider. The license must be at full clinical practice level to meet this requirement. A temporary license at the full clinical practice level is acceptable.

(ii) ***Professional certification requirement.*** When a state does not license a specific category of individual professional, certification by a Qualified Accreditation Organization, as defined in § 199.2, is required. Certification must be at full clinical practice level. A temporary certification at the full clinical practice level is acceptable.

(iii) ***Education, training and experience requirement.*** The Director, OCHAMPUS, or designee, may establish for each category or type of provider allowed by this paragraph (c) specific education, training, and experience requirements as necessary to promote the delivery of services by fully qualified individuals.

(iv) ***Physician referral and supervision.*** When physician referral and supervision is a prerequisite for CHAMPUS cost-sharing of the services of a provider authorized under this paragraph (c), such referral and supervision means that the physicians must actually see the patient to evaluate and diagnose the condition to be treated prior to referring the beneficiary to another provider and that the referring physician provides ongoing oversight of the course of referral related treatment throughout the period during which the beneficiary is being treated in response to the referral. Written contemporaneous documentation of the referring physician's basis for referral and ongoing communication between the referring and treating provider regarding the oversight of the treatment rendered as a result of the referral must meet all requirements for medical records established by this part. Referring physician supervision does not require physical location on the premises of the treating provider or at the site of treatment.

NOTE: **Emphasis** has been added to some text to delineate section headings.

# Appendix E

# Excerpts from Army Regulation 40–68: Selected Subsections Regarding the Scope of Practice and Supervision of Licensed Counselors

### 7–6. Behavioral health practitioner

. . . .

*c. Scope of practice.* Individuals will practice within the guidelines of their respective State licensing boards as LPCs [Licensed Professional Counselors] (or equivalent) or, if offered by their State, a license for master's-level psychology graduates such as psychological associate or licensed mental health provider. Behavioral health practitioners adhere to the State LPC or psychology licensing board's code of ethics and conduct. Specific clinical privileges are granted based upon training, experience, and competency. In general, behavioral health practitioners will—

(1) Conduct screening evaluations, utilizing information from clinical interviews, nonpsychometric tests, and collateral sources, as appropriate.

(2) Determine a provisional diagnosis according to the American Psychiatric Association Diagnostic and Statistical Manual of Mental Disorders.

(3) Provide individual and group behavioral health treatment within the scope of practice/privileges granted.

(4) Manage the behavioral health care of patients and refer those having needs beyond their scope of practice.

(5) Serve as collaborator in human behavioral issues with, and consultant to, community agencies, health care providers, and organizational leaders.

*d. Supervision.*

(1) Master's level graduates who have recently (within the past year) obtained a master's level license such as an LPC or psychological associate license, will be fully supervised during their first year of employment as a behavioral health practitioner.

(2) LPCs or psychological associates with 2 or more years' experience (after attaining licensure), will receive general supervision, according to the individual's level of competence, as assessed by his/her supervisor.

(3) LPCs or psychological associates with more than 2 years' experience and with post-master's work leading to a specialty degree, will require supervision in their specialty with difficult, high-risk cases, or for cases in which one or more of the patient's problems fall outside the scope of the counselor's specialty.

## REFERENCE

US Army. 2009. *Army Regulation 40–68. Medical Services. Clinical Quality Management.* Rapid Action Revision (RAR) Issue Date May 22, 2009. http://www.army.mil/usapa/epubs/pdf/r40_68.pdf. (Accessed October 3, 2009).

# Appendix F

# Case Summary Illustrating the Complexity of Mental Health Issues in the Military Population

*Kathryn Basham, PhD, LICSW*

The committee's report notes that special challenges are associated with the diagnosis of and treatment for mental health problems in a military population. This case summary illustrates the complexity of intersecting physical, psychological, and psychosocial issues that affect returning service members and their families. Even with sound resilience, many veterans and their families may still face a wide array of covarying diagnoses and other daunting conditions and challenges.

Case summaries are used as a teaching tool in clinical practice. This case[1] focuses on an identified individual client (patient) but should be viewed in the context of his family and social environment. *The content has been constructed as a composite clinical case; it is a fictitious account written for illustrative purposes only.*

## IDENTIFYING INFORMATION

Sgt. Carlos Arrozo, a 30-year-old Army veteran, returned from his 12-month tour of duty in Iraq 11 months ago. He worked as a communication specialist in charge of alerting convoys of transports to potential danger. On return to the United States, he received a medical

[1]The case was adapted and expanded from a clinical vignette contained in Basham (2009).

discharge based on his physical injuries and mental health injuries of posttraumatic stress disorder (PTSD) and major depression. He suffered second-degree and third-degree burns and a broken pelvis as a result of an improvised explosive device (IED) blast that killed two of his fellow soldiers.

Sgt. Arrozo lives with his 29-year-old wife of 10 years and his three young children—7, 5, and 2 years old—in a small city in North Carolina. After completing his high-school education focused on technical training, he enlisted in the Army, where he has served for the last 10 years. The family has a middle-income socioeconomic status. Maria Arrozo typically works on a part-time basis as a physical therapist. Both partners and their children are bilingual and speak Spanish and English interchangeably at home. The parents and children rely on their Catholic spiritual community as a source of hope, healing, and social support.

## PRESENTING ISSUES

### Individual

In the last two months, Sgt. Arrozo described pervasive anxiety, insomnia, nightmares, a fear of crowds, and flashbacks. One flashback occurred while he was driving with his wife to the grocery store. As they drove along a major highway in the middle lane, Sgt. Arrozo maintained his 60-mph speed until he saw a young adolescent boy leaning over the edge of a bridge that traversed the highway just 30 ft ahead. Knowing that the only thing he could do was continue forward, Sgt. Arrozo started to hyperventilate, sweat profusely, and increase his speed on the highway from 60 to 70 to 80 to 90 mph as he screamed to Maria to duck and take cover under the dashboard. As they sped frantically beneath the bridge, Maria screamed out in terror for Carlos to stop the car. Neither of them understood that this flashback was triggered by odors of gasoline and burning rubber, which were reminiscent of a traumatic incident involving a burning truck in Iraq. He fears remaining jobless and incapable of locating work in his field of communication. Worries about the possibility of a divorce from his wife plague him regularly.

Sgt. Arrozo also struggles with obsessional thoughts related to his guilt of surviving an IED blast that killed his fellow soldiers. He feels "dead to the world and deserving of death." Deep feelings of shame overwhelm him as he recalls "accidentally killing a helpless young child" in the course of the melee after an explosion. He suffers headaches, irritability, poor attention span, and poor concentration. Four months ago, he cried when his daughter Ana screamed hysterically after his futile attempt to pick her up to kiss her hello. He has not cried since. Every few hours, he experiences uncomfortable tingling and pain surrounding the newly grafted skin on his neck and arms.

Although previously an avid reader, Sgt. Arrozo cannot sit still to read or concentrate for more than 2 minutes. Most of the time, he feels alternately "tense, nauseated, agitated, irritable, enraged, and numb." He has trouble falling asleep, awakens fitfully throughout the night, and suffers nightmares and grogginess in the morning. He drinks eight beers with his buddies four or five times a week but is unconcerned about his alcohol intake.

## Family Psychosocial Issues

His wife, Maria, reported intense fear of her husband's "rage storms," describing him as "worked up, very loud, accusatory, and threatening to destroy everything in the house." She has warned him that if he fails to seek help, she will leave him and take the children to another state, and she has done that at least twice in the last 2 months. She has been experiencing insomnia, emotional volatility, and pervasive anxiety. The second-grade school teacher called the Arrozos about 7-year-old Antonio, who has started to talk back to the teacher and bully two of the smaller, quiet children in class. Delia, 5 years old, refuses to attend school and has started to wet her bed in recent weeks; Ana, 2 years old, alternates between playing joyfully and clinging anxiously to her mother's legs when her father enters the room.

## Developmental History

Developmental milestones appear to have been met adequately with no indication of childhood neglect or abuse. Elements of competence and resilience are noted in Sgt. Arrozo's academic success, diverse network of friends, and athletic prowess developed throughout his childhood and adult years. When Sgt. Arrozo turned 8 years old, his beloved mother died of ovarian cancer. The family arranged for a very hasty funeral and had little opportunity to share their mourning. Since her death, Sgt. Arrozo has seldom cried in response to his loss.

Shortly afterward his mother's death, his father married a woman who did not assume an active step-mothering role, and this contributed to Sgt. Arrozo's sadness and deep sense of abandonment. Early on, he coped with his losses through sublimation in relation to his studies and athletics. Although he and his immediate family live several hundred miles away from his father and siblings, he maintains regular contact with them by telephone and e-mail. He also communicates regularly with his extended family in Puerto Rico.

### Family History

Reared in Puerto Rico until the age of 6 years, Sgt. Arrozo moved with his parents and four siblings to the mainland in time for him to start elementary school. Although many Puerto Rican families lived in their community in the southeastern United States and provided strong social support, Sgt. Arrozo's family suffered discrimination and financial hardship. His wife, Maria, was the eldest of four children of parents who moved from Puerto Rico during their childhood years. They lived in an affluent urban community in the Northeast, where she and her siblings pursued college educations. The two families share the importance of sustaining family connections, valuing education and productivity and emphasizing the well-being of children.

### Mental Status in Process

Sgt. Arrozo appears to be fit and muscular, and he walks quickly and stiffly. His posture is noticeably rigid and upright in contrast with his casual, although clean and tidy, clothing that conceals any signs of the scarring covering his neck and arms. He is fluent in English and Spanish and speaks in a clear, coherent, and logical manner. Labile affect ranges from anxiety to sadness, despondency, irritation, agitation, and rage—all revealed in the course of 30-minute period. There is no evidence of hallucinations, delusions, or other symptoms related to psychosis.

## BIOPSYCHOSOCIAL ASSESSMENT

Sgt. Arrozo struggled with a complex set of physical, psychological, and psychosocial issues, which both influenced and were affected by interactions with his wife and family. Although they interrelate in a reciprocal manner, I will differentiate the various diagnoses and conditions of concern.

First, in the physical "bio" realm, he suffered pain and tingling in the aftermath of his treatment for second-degree burns. Insomnia persisted with pain and stiffness related to his healing pelvis. His expressions of irritability, headaches, and difficulties with balance, memory, and concentration are associated with the mild traumatic brain injury (TBI) that he sustained during an IED blast. This assessment was concluded 6 months after the start of treatment. Symptoms of irritability, poor memory, limited concentration, and emotional lability are also suggestive of alcohol abuse. Sgt. Arrozo meets the criteria of the *Diagnostic and Statistical Manual, Fourth Edition, Text Revision (DSM-IV-TR)* for substance abuse with failure to fulfill home and work obligations within the preceding year. Insomnia may be related to depression, pain, or substance abuse.

Second, in the realm of mental health "psycho" challenges, Sgt. Arrozo meets the criteria of major depression: depressed mood and markedly diminished interest in most activities, insomnia, psychomotor agitation, fatigue, inappropriate guilt, and diminished concentration. In addition to those symptoms of clinical depression, Sgt. Arrozo has suffered traumatic grief in response to the loss of his two beloved buddies during an IED blast. Because his job involves detection of potential hazards, he assumed major responsibility for the deaths of his friends. Compounding his profound grief and loss was the plaguing awareness that he had killed a young child during the melee that followed the same IED blast. He could not forgive himself and suffered profound guilt. Earlier unresolved grief related to the premature loss of his mother to cancer was reactivated after the untimely, traumatic deaths of his buddies and the Iraqi child.

Sgt. Arrozo also meets the criteria for PTSD with a full array of presenting issues related to the three clusters of re-experiencing (e.g., nightmares and flashbacks), avoidance (e.g., distancing from driving and shopping centers, detachment from children, and retreat from family), and hyperarousal (e.g., emotional lability, rage storms, and irritability).

Third, in the "social" or "psychosocial" realm, Sgt. Arrozo faces imminent divorce while he and his wife struggle bitterly with poor communication, destructive verbal exchanges, and impulsive, rageful outbursts alternating with distancing and detachment. Each of the children is expressing emotional distress. Seven-year-old Antonio may be carrying some unresolved intergenerational grief projected by his father, who at the same age lost his mother to death from ovarian cancer. Like many children who suffer anxiety and depression, they express their feelings behaviorally through aggressive bullying and negativity. Delia may also be responding to the forces of secondary trauma that affect family members who live with a traumatized person. Her heightened anxiety, evidenced by her fears of separating to attend school, mirrors Sgt. Arrozo's intense fears engendered by the presence of her loud and agitated father. Sgt. Arrozo also worries about securing employment; in the meantime, the family suffers both financially and psychologically from accumulated stress.

## *DSM-IV-TR* DIAGNOSES

Axis I Posttraumatic stress disorder
Major depressive disorder
Substance abuse—alcohol

Axis II Deferred

Axis III Mild traumatic brain injury, skin grafts on neck and arms after second-degree and third-degree burns, healing from broken pelvis

Axis IV Severe stressors: deaths of his two combat buddies, marital separations and anticipated divorce, joblessness, financial pressures, distress for wife and children

Axis V Poor level of functioning (GAF score: 40) evidenced by disruptions in his physical and mental health, marriage, parenting, relationships with friends and family, job seeking

## TREATMENT PLAN

### Part I

When Sgt. Arrozo agreed to seek mental health assistance, his wife, Maria, telephoned to access a mental health provider authorized by TRICARE. After receiving the name of a licensed nonmedical mental health clinician, Sgt. Arrozo was invited to attend an individual session to embark on an assessment. After a 1-hour meeting, the preliminary diagnosis of PTSD and depression was established on the basis of his medical discharge. To help Sgt. Arrozo to experience rapid relief from his combat-related psychological injuries, the clinician referred him to a colleague for prolonged exposure therapy. Goals of that therapy included reduction in nightmares, reduction in flashbacks, and increased capacity to drive and shop. The clinician also recommended 1 hour of individual psychotherapy each week to address the symptoms of depression. The treatment plan included psychoeducation related to PTSD and depression and the use of cognitive–behavioral therapy (CBT) skills to track depressed moods and challenge faulty attributions through journaling.

Treatment goals included reduction in negative self-attributions and increased recognition of PTSD-related symptoms and behaviors. Although his general practitioner had prescribed Zoloft to address symptoms of PTSD and depression, the mental health clinician never sought consultation or collaboration with that physician. Sgt. Arrozo could not concentrate on his daily writing assignments and felt ashamed of his incapacity to improve. After 3 weeks of the combined treatment, flooding of emotions overwhelmed Sgt. Arrozo, and he decompensated, reporting intense suicidal thoughts several times throughout the day. He terminated his therapy.

### Clinical Impasse

Was Sgt. Arrozo a failure, or were there unintended iatrogenic effects related to the absence of a thorough biopsychosocial assessment and differential diagnosis? Was there a failure on the part of the clinician to attend to the totality of this veteran's struggles in addition to exploring his resilience in his social context? Apparently, his undiagnosed mild TBI interfered with his benefiting from a cognitive-behavioral method that requires reasonably sound cognitive functioning. Ignoring the presence of an alcohol-abuse problem prevented the clinician and Sgt. Arrozo from addressing the adverse effects of alcohol on his overall functioning. Did the PTSD-related issues of sleep disturbance, irritability, and hyperarousal also mimic symptoms that are associated with alcohol abuse? How did his alcohol intake interact with the use of an antidepressant and pain medication? Did it negate potential positive effects? Was the pharmacologic intervention the most effective plan, given the complexity of his conditions?

While ignoring cultural responsiveness, did the clinician explore the sociocultural meanings and stigma related to mental health problems for Sgt. Arrozo and his wife? Was consideration given to assessing social and community supports (e.g., extended family, church, work colleagues, and friendship network) to facilitate the family's engagement in an effective treatment plan? Finally, the absence of attunement to the volatile relationship between the marital partners and between the parents and the children set the stage for increasing decompensation and further destabilization. Was a risk assessment completed? Are there aspects of intimate-partner violence that are concealed? Are Sgt. Arrozo, Delia, and Ana expressing symptoms of secondary trauma evidenced by signs of heightened insecurity, anxiety, and aggression?

## Part II

After Sgt. Arrozo ended his treatment precipitously, he felt very wary of any potential usefulness of mental health treatment. Yet, when each of his children's teachers called to express serious concerns about their emotional well-being, Sgt. Arrozo and his wife registered alarm and decided to work with another mental health professional. Once again, they pursued a referral recommended by TRICARE. This time, a female nonmedical licensed mental health clinician responded to Sgt. Arrozo and invited him to participate in a consultation session to discuss possible next steps. Although reluctant, Sgt. Arrozo was reassured to hear that he had not failed in his treatment. Instead, this clinician needed to explore a full biopsychosocial assessment that addressed many of his life challenges and supports.

Collaborative consultative relationships and carefully selected referrals were initiated with a network of providers, including a general practitioner, a psychiatrist, a vocational counselor, a rehabilitation counselor, school counselors for the children, a couple/family therapist, and a support group facilitated by combat veterans. A phase-oriented trauma-based treatment plan was instituted in the first session that, early on, attended to issues of safety, stabilization, self-care, and establishing a context for change. Clinical case management emerged as a primary modality during this period of crisis as the clinician established a treatment plan involving a deftly coordinated and collaborative treatment plan. Individual supportive psychotherapy was offered to Sgt. Arrozo to explore the most effective ways to establish his self-care (vis-à-vis his symptoms of PTSD, depression, and substance abuse) and to restore connections with his family and his faith-based community. Motivational interviewing was introduced to engage Sgt. Arrozo in discussions that focused on the role that alcohol played in his life.

Treatment goals included demonstrating skills to reduce stress and anger, demonstrating skills in tolerating distress, applying stress reduction and relaxation techniques, communicating directly with his wife and children, recognizing feeling states that are associated with a traumatic stress response, recognizing the effects of alcohol on his daily functioning, developing a plan to work with a rehabilitation counselor in relation to his TBI. Within 4 months, progress toward all those goals was noted. Only when safety had been established, both individually and in the marital relationship, could Sgt. Arrozo engage with cognitive processing treatment, which allowed him to address the legacies of his combat trauma experiences in a titrated, balanced manner. That led to his greater understanding of the after-effects of combat trauma and how attachments and relationships can be dismantled by wartime combat. As he slowly reestablished his trust in his relationships with his wife and children, he recognized how a solid base of family and emotional support proved essential as well. Couple therapy focused on enhancing communication, addressing power differentials and shifting coparenting roles, and finally minimizing the potential for intimate-partner violence. With a more secure base, he started to address his profound grief associated with the losses of his buddies, the Iraqi child, and his mother. With a stronger scaffolding of coping measures in place, Sgt. Arrozo was able to bear the intensity of his mourning. As he discussed his experience of profound guilt, the clinician and Sgt. Arrozo explored his lapsed faith and a cultural belief that his warrior behavior represented a betrayal to family and community. With those complex issues openly addressed, Sgt. Arrozo gradually reported relief from deep sadness and pessimism while developing a more textured understanding of his combat role.

In summary, this sample treatment case reveals both the depth of pain suffered by Sgt. Arrozo and his family and their distinct resilience that enabled them to thrive and reclaim healthy, more positive and productive lives together. Such progress is noteworthy and can serve as an exemplar for many other veterans and their families who need and deserve high-quality mental health care. Although the first treatment plan missed important dimensions of Sgt. Arrozo's presenting issues, the second course of treatment proved far more successful. That phase-oriented treatment plan stressed attunement to the therapeutic alliance, cultural responsiveness, knowledge and skills based on relevant evidence-based practice models, continuing collaboration and consultation, and flexibility to assess and treat a complex, multidimensioned set of conditions and challenges. To promote similar favorable outcomes in practice with service members and their families, each clinician needs to be prepared with satisfactory education from an accredited academic institution, ample supervised clinical experience with a broad array of clients, and certification, licensure, and privileging within a scope of practice. Given the serious adverse consequences of failed treatment, we must be vigilant in our evaluations of potential mental health clinicians.

## REFERENCE

Basham K. 2009. Commentary on the keynote lecture presented by Dr. Jonathan Shay, Friday, June 27, 2008, titled "The trials of homecoming: Odysseus returns from Iraq/Afghanistan, and additional reflections." *Smith College Studies in Social Work* 79(3&4):299-309.

# Appendix G

# State Laws and Regulations Regarding the Practice of Counselors as of November 2009

| State | Credentials[a] | Definition | Educational Requirements[b] |
|---|---|---|---|
| Alabama | Licensed Professional Counselor | A person who renders professional counseling services in private practice to individuals, groups, organizations, corporations, institutions, government agencies, or the general public | Master's degree or higher in counseling from a CACREP- or CORE-accredited program or its equivalent at a regionally accredited institution, with at least 48 graduate semester hours |
| Alaska | Licensed Professional Counselor | | Master's degree or higher in counseling or a related field (including psychology, marital and family therapy, social work, and applied behavioral science) from a CACREP-accredited program or its equivalent, with at least 60 graduate semester hours in counseling, including coursework in eight core subjects |

| Clinical-Experience Requirements | Licensing Requirements[c] | License Renewal and Continuing Education | Independent Practice? | Health-Insurance Coverage[d] |
|---|---|---|---|---|
| 3,000 hours of supervised experience in professional counseling under a board-approved supervisor; 1,000 hours of the required experience may be subtracted for every 15 graduate semester hours obtained beyond the master's degree | Applicant must be at least 19 years old, have a master's degree focused primarily in professional counseling, have completed the required hours of professional experience, have passed the NCE | License renewal every 2 years; requires 40 contact hours, 6 hours of continuing education in ethics | Yes—assessment, diagnosis, treatment planning, individual and group counseling | |
| 3,000 hours of supervised experience in professional counseling, including 1,000 hours of direct client contact, 100 hours of face-to-face supervision under an LPC or other licensed mental health professional (can be by telephone or electronic means because of remote location of counselor) | Applicant must be at least 18 years old, have a master's or doctoral degree in counseling, have completed the required number of hours of professional experience, have passed the NCE | License renewal every 2 years; requires 40 contact hours | Yes—assessment, diagnosis, treatment planning, individual and group counseling | |

*continued*

| State | Credentials[a] | Definition | Educational Requirements[b] |
|---|---|---|---|
| Arizona | Licensed Professional Counselor | | Master's degree or higher in counseling or a related field from a CACREP- or CORE-accredited program that includes at least 60 semester hours and coursework in 14 content subjects |
| Arkansas | Licensed Professional Counselor; Licensed Associate Counselor | LAC: an applicant with less than 3 years of post–master's-level supervision experience if all other requirements have been met | Master's degree or higher in counseling with at least 60 semester hours in a program that reflects the CACREP or CORE curriculum, from a regionally accredited institution |

| Clinical-Experience Requirements | Licensing Requirements[c] | License Renewal and Continuing Education | Independent Practice? | Health-Insurance Coverage[d] |
|---|---|---|---|---|
| 2 years or 3,200 hours of full-time post-master's supervised work experience in psychotherapy, including assessment, diagnosis, and treatment, with 100 hours of clinical supervision and 1,600 hours of direct client contact | Applicant must have successfully completed all core courses required for a master's degree from an accredited program, have the required number of professional experience hours, have passed the NCE, NCMHCE, or CRCE | License renewal every 2 years; requires 40 contact hours, 3 hours of continuing education in behavioral health ethics or mental health law, 3 hours in cultural competence and diversity | Yes—assessment, diagnosis, treatment planning, individual and group counseling | |
| 3 years or 3,000 hours of post-master's supervised experience under a board-approved supervisor (1 year = 1,000 hours); 1 year of experience may be gained for each 30 semester hours earned beyond a master's degree (up to 2 years) | Applicant must have received graduate training in higher education primarily related to professional counseling, have completed the required number of years of professional supervised experience, have passed the NCE and an oral examination | License renewal every 2 years; requires 24 contact hours, 2 hours of continuing education in ethics | Yes, LPC only—assessment, diagnosis, treatment planning, individual and group counseling | Mandated coverage, mandated offering, any willing provider |

*continued*

| State | Credentials[a] | Definition | Educational Requirements[b] |
|---|---|---|---|
| California | Licensed Professional Clinical Counselor | | For those grandfathered in or beginning graduate study before August 1, 2012, a master's or doctoral degree from an accredited or approved institution with 48 semester hours in a program that is counseling or psychotherapy in content; for those beginning graduate study after August 1, 2012, a 60-semester-unit master's or doctoral degree from an accredited or approved institution that is counseling or psychotherapy in content |
| Colorado | Licensed Professional Counselor | | Master's degree or higher in professional counseling from a CACREP-accredited program or regionally accredited institution with 48 semester hours, including coursework in core subjects and a practicum or internship |

| Clinical-Experience Requirements | Licensing Requirements[c] | License Renewal and Continuing Education | Independent Practice? | Health-Insurance Coverage[d] |
|---|---|---|---|---|
| At least 3,000 post-degree hours of supervised experience by an LPC, LMFT, LCSW, licensed psychologist, or licensed psychiatrist over a period of at least 2 years, including at least 1,750 hours of direct counseling with individuals or groups in a clinical mental health–counseling setting and 150 hours in a hospital or community mental health setting | Applicant must have completed all degree and clinical experience requirements, have obtained a passing score on examinations approved by the board, probably the NCE, the NCMHCE, and a California jurisprudence and ethics examination | Licenses will be issued beginning January 1, 2011, and must be renewed annually or biannually; requires 18 hours of approved continuing education annually | Yes—assessment, diagnosis, treatment planning, individual and group counseling | |
| 2 years or 2,000 hours of post-master's practice in applied psychotherapy under board-approved supervision, including 100 hours of supervision, of which 70 must be individual supervision | Applicant must be at least 21 years old, have a master's degree in professional counseling, have completed the necessary years of post-master's practice, have passed the NCE and the Colorado jurisprudence examination | License renewal every 2 years; no continuing-education requirement | Yes—assessment, diagnosis, treatment planning, individual and group counseling | |

*continued*

| State | Credentials[a] | Definition | Educational Requirements[b] |
|---|---|---|---|
| Connecticut | Licensed Professional Counselor | | Master's degree or higher in counseling or related mental health field from a regionally accredited institution consisting of at least 60 semester hours, completion of required coursework, and a sixth-year degree in counseling |

| Clinical-Experience Requirements | Licensing Requirements[c] | License Renewal and Continuing Education | Independent Practice? | Health-Insurance Coverage[d] |
|---|---|---|---|---|
| 1 year or 3,000 hours of post-master's supervised experience in professional counseling with at least 100 hours of direct supervision | Applicant must have a master's or doctoral degree in social work, marriage and family therapy, counseling, psychology, or a related mental health field; have completed the required number of hours of postgraduate professional experience; have passed the NCE or NCMHCE | License renewal annually; requires 15 contact hours | Yes—assessment, diagnosis, treatment planning, individual and group counseling | Mandated coverage |

*continued*

| State | Credentials[a] | Definition | Educational Requirements[b] |
|---|---|---|---|
| Delaware | Licensed Professional Counselor of Mental Health | | Master's degree or higher, including at least 48 semester hours |
| District of Columbia | Licensed Professional Counselor | | Master's degree in counseling or a related field, including 60 graduate semester hours and coursework in 10 core subjects (including a practicum or internship) |

| Clinical-Experience Requirements | Licensing Requirements[c] | License Renewal and Continuing Education | Independent Practice? | Health-Insurance Coverage[d] |
|---|---|---|---|---|
| 3,000 hours of full-time clinical professional counseling experience within a 4-year period, of which 1,600 hours must be professional direct supervision (including 100 hours of face-to-face supervision); 30 graduate semester hours or more beyond a master's degree may be substituted for 1 year or 1,600 hours of required experience | Applicant must have a graduate degree, have completed the required number of professional experience hours, have passed the NCE or NCMHCE, be certified by the NBCC as a CCMHC or by another national mental health specialty certifying organization | License renewal every 2 years; requires 40 contact hours | Yes—assessment, diagnosis, treatment planning, individual and group counseling | |
| 2 years or 3,500 hours of post-master's supervised professional counseling experience, including 200 hours under an LPC and 100 hours of "immediate supervision"; remaining hours can be under supervision of any licensed mental health professional | Applicant must have a master's degree, have completed the required number of professional experience hours, have passed the NCE, NCMHCE, or CRCE | License renewal every 2 years; no continuing-education requirement | Yes—assessment, diagnosis, treatment planning, individual and group counseling | |

*continued*

| State | Credentials[a] | Definition | Educational Requirements[b] |
|---|---|---|---|
| Florida | Licensed Mental Health Counselor | | Master's degree or higher from a CACREP-accredited mental health counseling program, including 60 semester hours, a course in human sexuality, and a course in substance abuse OR a master's degree or higher from a program related to the practice of mental health counseling from an accredited institution, including 60 semester hours, 12 specific content subjects, and 1,000 hours of supervised practicum, internship, or field experience, AND FOR BOTH OPTIONS completion of an 8-hour laws-and-rules course and a 2-hour prevention-of-medical-errors course |

| Clinical-Experience Requirements | Licensing Requirements[c] | License Renewal and Continuing Education | Independent Practice? | Health-Insurance Coverage[d] |
|---|---|---|---|---|
| 2 years of supervised post-master's clinical experience in mental health counseling, consisting of at least 1,500 hours of providing psychotherapy face to face with clients and at least 100 hours of face-to-face supervision under an LMHC or equivalent (50 hours of which can be group supervision) | Applicant must have a master's degree, have completed the clinical supervision requirements and the additional courses on laws and rules and on prevention of medical errors, have passed the NCMHCE | License renewal every 2 years; requires 30 contact hours, 2 hours of continuing education in prevention of medical errors, 3 hours in ethics and boundary issues; every third renewal requires 2 hours of training on domestic violence | Yes—assessment, diagnosis, treatment planning, individual and group counseling | Mandated offering |

*continued*

| State | Credentials[a] | Definition | Educational Requirements[b] |
| --- | --- | --- | --- |
| Georgia | Licensed Professional Counselor | | Master's degree or higher in a program primarily counseling in content or in applied psychology from an institution accredited by a regional body recognized by CHEA, including specific coursework and a supervised practicum or internship of at least 300 hours |

| Clinical-Experience Requirements | Licensing Requirements[c] | License Renewal and Continuing Education | Independent Practice? | Health-Insurance Coverage[d] |
|---|---|---|---|---|
| 4 years or 2,400 hours of supervised post-master's experience in professional counseling, with at least 120 hours of supervision and at least 2 years of supervision provided by an LPC OR 3 years or 1,800 hours of supervised post-master's experience in professional counseling (2 years of which must be under the supervision of an LPC), at least 90 hours of supervision, a supervised counseling practicum or internship of at least 300 hours as part of the graduate program | Applicant must have a master's or doctoral degree in a field related to professional counseling, have completed all clinical experience requirements, have passed the NCE | License renewal every 2 years; requires 35 contact hours, 5 hours of continuing education in ethics | Yes—assessment, treatment planning, individual and group counseling | |

*continued*

| State | Credentials[a] | Definition | Educational Requirements[b] |
|---|---|---|---|
| Hawaii | Licensed Mental Health Counselor | | Master's degree or higher in counseling or an allied field related to the practice of mental health counseling with at least 48 semester hours, including coursework in core subjects, from an accredited institution; program must include two academic terms (of at least 3 semester hours each) of supervised mental health practicum intern experience in a mental health–counseling setting with at least 300 hours of supervised client contact under a licensed supervisor |

| Clinical-Experience Requirements | Licensing Requirements[c] | License Renewal and Continuing Education | Independent Practice? | Health-Insurance Coverage[d] |
|---|---|---|---|---|
| 2 years or 3,000 hours of post-master's experience in the practice of mental health counseling with 100 hours of face-to-face clinical supervision under a licensed supervisor (experience should be completed in at least 2 years and no more than 4 years) | Applicant must have a master's or doctoral degree, have completed all required hours of supervised clinical experience, have passed the NCE | License renewal every 3 years; no continuing-education requirement | Yes—assessment, diagnosis, treatment planning, individual and group therapy | |

continued

| State | Credentials[a] | Definition | Educational Requirements[b] |
|---|---|---|---|
| Idaho | Licensed Clinical Professional Counselor; Licensed Professional Counselor | | Master's degree or higher in a counseling field from an accredited institution with 60 semester hours and completion of a 6-semester-hour advanced counseling practicum |

| Clinical-Experience Requirements | Licensing Requirements[c] | License Renewal and Continuing Education | Independent Practice? | Health-Insurance Coverage[d] |
|---|---|---|---|---|
| LCPC: must hold a valid LPC license and have 2 years or 2,000 hours of supervised direct client-contact experience accumulated after licensure, 1,000 hours of which are under the supervision of an LCPC, with at least 1 hour of face-to-face, one-on-one supervision for every 30 hours of direct client contact; must also successfully complete a diagnostic-evaluation graduate course or equivalent training or experience; LPC: 1,000 hours of supervised experience in counseling, with 400 hours of direct client contact and at least 1 hour of face-to-face supervision for every 20 hours of experience | LCPC must have passed the NCMHCE; LPC must have passed the NCE | License renewal annually; requires 20 contact hours, 3 hours of continuing education in ethics | Yes—assessment, treatment planning, individual and group counseling | |

*continued*

| State | Credentials[a] | Definition | Educational Requirements[b] |
|---|---|---|---|
| Illinois | Licensed Clinical Professional Counselor; Licensed Professional Counselor | LCPC: a person who holds a license authorizing independent practice of clinical professional counseling in private practice; LPC: a person who holds a license authorizing the practice of professional counseling | LCPC: master's degree or higher in counseling or a related field from a regionally accredited college or university OR current CCMHC credential issued by NBCC; LPC: master's degree or higher in professional counseling or related field, including at least 48 semester hours, from an accredited institution (CACREP- and CORE-accredited programs in professional counseling are approved for both LCPCs and LPCs) |

| Clinical-Experience Requirements | Licensing Requirements[c] | License Renewal and Continuing Education | Independent Practice? | Health-Insurance Coverage[d] |
|---|---|---|---|---|
| LCPC: 2 years or 3,000 hours of full-time postgraduate supervised employment or experience working as a clinical professional counselor in a professional capacity under the direction of a qualified supervisor, of which 1,920 hours must be in direct face-to-face service to clients (1 year = maximum of 1,680 hours, including 960 hours of direct face-to-face service to clients); LPC with master's degree: not required to obtain additional experience for licensure | LCPC must have passed the NCE and NCMHCE or ECCP or CRCE; LPC must have passed the NCE or CRCE | License renewal every 2 years; requires 30 contact hours | Yes—assessment, treatment planning, individual and group counseling | Mandated offering |

*continued*

| State | Credentials[a] | Definition | Educational Requirements[b] |
|---|---|---|---|
| Indiana | Licensed Mental Health Counselor | | Master's degree or higher in a field related to mental health counseling (including counseling, clinical social work, psychology, human services, human development, and family relations) from a CACREP- or CORE-accredited, or equivalent, program from a regionally accredited institution, including at least 60 semester hours in counseling in 12 content subjects and completion of a practicum (100 hours), internship (600 hours), and advanced internship (300 hours) with at least 100 hours of face-to-face supervision |

| Clinical-Experience Requirements | Licensing Requirements[c] | License Renewal and Continuing Education | Independent Practice? | Health-Insurance Coverage[d] |
|---|---|---|---|---|
| 3,000 hours of postgraduate clinical experience over a 21-month period, including 100 hours of face-to-face supervision under an LMHC or equivalent supervisor | Applicant must have completed all degree and clinical-experience requirements, have passed the NCMHCE | License renewal every 2 years; requires 40 contact hours (20 hours per year), 2 hours of continuing education in ethics and professional conduct (1 hour per year) | Yes—assessment, diagnosis, treatment planning, and individual and group counseling | |

*continued*

| State | Credentials[a] | Definition | Educational Requirements[b] |
|---|---|---|---|
| Iowa | Licensed Mental Health Counselor | | Master's degree or higher in counseling from a CACREP- or CORE-accredited program, or equivalent with at least 60 graduate semester hours, at a regionally accredited institution OR current CCMHC credential issued by NBCC |

| Clinical-Experience Requirements | Licensing Requirements[c] | License Renewal and Continuing Education | Independent Practice? | Health-Insurance Coverage[d] |
|---|---|---|---|---|
| 2 years of full-time postgraduate supervised work experience in mental health counseling, with 2,000 hours of face-to-face mental health counseling; at least 100 of the 200 hours of clinical supervision must be individual supervision | Applicant must have completed all degree and clinical-experience requirements, have passed the NCE, NCMHCE, or CRCE | License renewal every 2 years; requires 40 contact hours, 2 hours of continuing education in child-abuse identification and reporting training for counselors who treat children, 2 hours of dependent-adult–abuse identification and reporting training for counselors who work with adults | Yes—assessment, diagnosis, treatment planning, individual and group counseling | |

*continued*

| State | Credentials[a] | Definition | Educational Requirements[b] |
|---|---|---|---|
| Kansas | Licensed Clinical Professional Counselor; Licensed Professional Counselor | LPC: a person who may practice under the direction of an LCPC; LCPC: a person licensed to provide mental health services as an independent practitioner and whose license allows diagnosis of and treatment for mental disorders. | LCPC: in addition to or as part of graduate degree, completion of 15 credit hours supporting diagnosis of and treatment for mental disorders with use of the *DSM* and completion of graduate-level supervised clinical practicum of professional experience; LPC: master's degree in counseling from a university approved by the board, including 45 graduate semester hours in 10 core categories and a total of 60 graduate semester hours (including supervised practicum) |
| Kentucky | Licensed Professional Clinical Counselor | | Master's degree or higher in professional counseling or a related field from a regionally accredited institution with at least 60 semester hours in nine specified content subjects and a 400-hour practicum or internship |

| Clinical-Experience Requirements | Licensing Requirements[c] | License Renewal and Continuing Education | Independent Practice? | Health-Insurance Coverage[d] |
|---|---|---|---|---|
| LCPC: must be licensed as an LPC or meet all requirements to be licensed as an LPC and have 2 years or 4,000 hours of supervised clinical professional counseling experience under an approved clinical training plan, including 1,500 hours of direct client contact and 150 hours of clinical supervision | LCPC must have passed the NCMHCE; LPC must have passed the NCE | License renewal every 2 years; requires 30 contact hours, 3 hours of continuing education in ethics, 6 hours related to the diagnosis and treatment of mental disorders | Yes—assessment, diagnosis, treatment planning, individual and group counseling | |
| 4,000 hours of post-master's experience in the practice of counseling under approved supervision, including 1,600 hours of direct counseling and 100 hours of individual, face-to-face clinical supervision | Applicant must have completed all degree and clinical-experience requirements, have passed the NCE | License renewal annually; requires 10 contact hours | Yes—assessment, diagnosis, treatment planning, individual and group counseling | |

*continued*

| State | Credentials[a] | Definition | Educational Requirements[b] |
|---|---|---|---|
| Louisiana | Licensed Professional Counselor | | Master's degree or higher in a program primarily professional mental health counseling in content from a regionally accredited institution with 48 semester hours and coursework in eight content subjects OR completion of a CACREP-accredited counseling program, which must include a supervised practicum (100 hours) and supervised internship (300 hours) in mental health counseling |

| Clinical-Experience Requirements | Licensing Requirements[c] | License Renewal and Continuing Education | Independent Practice? | Health-Insurance Coverage[d] |
|---|---|---|---|---|
| 2 years or 3,000 hours of post-master's supervised experience in professional mental health counseling under the clinical supervision of a board-approved supervisor to be completed in no more than 7 years and to include 1,900–2,900 hours of direct client contact in individual or group counseling, with a minimum of 100 hours of face-to-face supervision; 500 hours of supervised experience may be gained for each 30 graduate semester hours beyond a master's degree, but applicant must have at least 2,000 hours of supervised postgraduate experience | Applicant must be at least 21 years old and a resident of Louisiana, have completed all degree and clinical-experience requirements, have passed the NCE | License renewal every 2 years; requires 40 contact hours | Yes—assessment, diagnosis, treatment planning, individual and group counseling | Mandated offering |

*continued*

| State | Credentials[a] | Definition | Educational Requirements[b] |
|---|---|---|---|
| Maine | Licensed Clinical Professional Counselor; Licensed Professional Counselor | | LCPC: master's degree or higher from a CACREP-accredited program that consists of 60 semester hours or coursework in 10 core subjects, three additional subjects, and a practicum or internship of 900 hours;<br>LPC: master's degree or higher from a CACREP- or CORE-accredited program that consists of 48 semester hours or coursework in 10 core subjects and a practicum and internship of 600 hours |

| Clinical-Experience Requirements | Licensing Requirements[c] | License Renewal and Continuing Education | Independent Practice? | Health-Insurance Coverage[d] |
|---|---|---|---|---|
| LCPC: 2 years or 3,000 hours of post-master's supervised clinical counseling experience, including 1,500 hours of direct client contact and 100 hours of clinical supervision with an approved supervisor; LPC: 2 years or 2,000 hours of post-master's supervised counseling experience, including 1,000 hours of direct counseling and 67 hours of supervision under an approved supervisor | LCPC must have passed the NCMHCE; LPC must have passed the NCE | License renewal every 2 years; requires 55 contact hours | Yes, both LCPC and LPC—assessment, individual and group counseling; LCPC can diagnose, treat | Mandated offering |

continued

| State | Credentials[a] | Definition | Educational Requirements[b] |
|---|---|---|---|
| Maryland | Licensed Clinical Professional Counselor | | Master's degree or higher in a professional counseling or related field from an accredited institution with at least 60 graduate semester hours, including specific coursework in alcohol and drug-abuse counseling and supervised field experience OR doctoral degree with at least 90 graduate semester hours in counseling training |

| Clinical-Experience Requirements | Licensing Requirements[c] | License Renewal and Continuing Education | Independent Practice? | Health-Insurance Coverage[d] |
|---|---|---|---|---|
| For those with a master's degree: 3 years or 3,000 hours of supervised clinical experience in professional counseling (2 years or 2,000 hours must be post-master's clinical supervision), including 1,500 hours of face-to-face client contact and at least 100 hours of face-to-face clinical supervision under a board-approved supervisor; for those with a doctoral degree: 2 years or 2,000 hours of supervised clinical experience in professional counseling, 1 year or 1,000 hours of which must be postdoctorate and 1,000 hours face-to-face client contact, with at least 50 hours of face-to-face clinical supervision under a board-approved supervisor | Applicants must have completed all degree and clinical-experience requirements, have passed the NCE and Maryland Law Test on the Professional Counselors and Therapists Act | License renewal every 2 years; requires 40 contact hours | Yes—assessment, diagnosis, treatment planning, individual and group counseling | Mandated coverage |

continued

| State | Credentials[a] | Definition | Educational Requirements[b] |
|---|---|---|---|
| Massachusetts | Licensed Mental Health Counselor | | Master's degree in counseling or a related field from a regionally accredited institution with at least 60 graduate semester hours, including a minimum 48 semester hours in mental health counseling or a related field involving a practicum (100 hours), internship (600 hours), and coursework in 10 content subjects OR current CCMHC credential issued by NBCC |
| Michigan | Licensed Professional Counselor | | Master's degree or higher in professional counseling, including at least 48 semester hours from a program reflecting the CACREP curriculum and a 600-hour internship |

| Clinical-Experience Requirements | Licensing Requirements[c] | License Renewal and Continuing Education | Independent Practice? | Health-Insurance Coverage[d] |
|---|---|---|---|---|
| 2 years or 3,360 hours of full-time post-master's supervised clinical experience in mental health counseling, including 960 hours of direct client contact (250 hours of which may be group client contact) and 130 hours of supervision (75 hours of which must be individual supervision); hours do not include practicum and internship supervision requirements | Applicant must have a master's degree from an institution licensed in counseling education, have completed the required hours of supervised clinical experience, have passed the NCMHCE | License renewal every 2 years; requires 30 contact hours | Yes—assessment, diagnosis, treatment planning, individual and group counseling | Mandated coverage |
| 2 years or 3,000 hours of postdegree supervised counseling experience, including at least 100 hours under the immediate physical presence of the supervisor, who must be an LPC; 30 semester hours beyond the master's degree may be substituted for 1 year or 1,500 hours postdegree supervised experience (including 50 hours of immediate supervision) | Applicant must have a master's or doctoral degree in counseling or student personnel work from an approved program, have completed supervised counseling under a licensed professional counselor, have passed the NCE or CRCE | License renewal every 3 years; no continuing-education requirement | Yes—assessment, diagnosis, treatment planning, individual and group counseling | Any willing provider |

continued

| State | Credentials[a] | Definition | Educational Requirements[b] |
|---|---|---|---|
| Minnesota | Licensed Professional Clinical Counselor (new licensure tier as of August 2007); Licensed Professional Counselor | | LPCC: in addition to or as part of the graduate degree in counseling or a related field, completion of 24 graduate-level semester credits in six clinical content subjects; LPC: master's degree or higher in counseling or a related field from a CACREP-accredited program or regionally accredited institution, including at least 48 semester hours, at least 700 hours of supervised field experience in counseling, and coursework in 10 core content subjects |

| Clinical-Experience Requirements | Licensing Requirements[c] | License Renewal and Continuing Education | Independent Practice? | Health-Insurance Coverage[d] |
|---|---|---|---|---|
| LPCC: 4,000 hours of post-master's supervised professional practice in the clinical diagnosis and treatment of mental disorders in children and adults, including 1,800 hours of clinical client contact, with at least 50% under individual supervision; LPC: 1 year or 2,000 hours of post-master's supervised professional practice to be completed in no more than 3 years, including 100 hours of supervision under an LPC, licensed psychologist, or other qualified supervisor | Applicant must be at least 18 years old, have completed the required degree and clinical-experience requirements, have passed a national examination; LPCC must have passed the NCMHCE (or both the NCE and ECCP), have passed ethical, oral, and situational examinations; LPC must have passed the NCE | License renewal annually; requires 40 hours of continuing education and 12 graduate semester credits in counseling in the first 4 years of license or completion of the number of graduate credits sufficient to reach a combined total of 60 graduate semester credits between the degree program and this requirement | Yes, both LPCC and LPC—assessment, diagnosis, treatment planning, individual and group counseling | |

continued

| State | Credentials[a] | Definition | Educational Requirements[b] |
|---|---|---|---|
| Mississippi | Licensed Professional Counselor | | Master's degree or educational specialist's degree in counselor education or a related program from a regionally accredited program with 60 semester hours and completion of coursework in 10 content subjects OR doctoral degree primarily in counseling, guidance, or related counseling field from a regionally accredited program |

| Clinical-Experience Requirements | Licensing Requirements[c] | License Renewal and Continuing Education | Independent Practice? | Health-Insurance Coverage[d] |
|---|---|---|---|---|
| 2 years or 3,500 hours of supervised counseling experience in a clinical setting, of which at least 1,750 must be post-master's experience and at least 1,167 must be direct counseling service to clients, with at least 100 hours of supervision (50 hours may be group supervision) under an LPC designated as a board-approved qualified supervisor | Applicant must be at least 21 years old, be a resident of Mississippi, have completed all educational and experience requirements, have passed the NCE | License renewal annually; requires 12 contact hours, 3 hours of continuing education in ethics or legal issues | Yes—assessment, diagnosis, treatment planning, individual and group counseling | Mandated coverage |

*continued*

| State | Credentials[a] | Definition | Educational Requirements[b] |
|---|---|---|---|
| Missouri | Licensed Professional Counselor | | Master's degree or higher in counseling, counseling psychology, clinical psychology, or school psychology from a regionally accredited institution with at least 48 semester hours reflecting the CACREP or CORE curriculum and a practicum, internship, or field experience consisting of 6 semester hours in the practice of counseling |

| Clinical-Experience Requirements | Licensing Requirements[c] | License Renewal and Continuing Education | Independent Practice? | Health-Insurance Coverage[d] |
|---|---|---|---|---|
| 2 years or 3,000 hours of post-master's continuous counseling experience to be completed within 60 months; 1,200 hours must be direct client contact, with 15 hours of supervised counseling per week, of which 1 hour per week is face-to-face supervision (30 hours of post-master's study may be substituted for 1,500 hours of supervised experience); if person obtained a doctorate or specialist's degree, 1 year or 1,500 hours of counseling experience to be completed within 36 months, including 600 hours of direct client contact, 15 hours of supervised counseling per week, and 1 hour of face-to-face supervision per week; all supervision must be under an LPC or licensed psychologist or psychiatrist | Applicant must have a master's or doctoral degree from an approved program, have completed supervised counseling, have passed the NCE | License renewal every 2 years; requires 40 contact hours | Yes—assessment, diagnosis, treatment planning, individual and group counseling | Mandated offering |

*continued*

| State | Credentials[a] | Definition | Educational Requirements[b] |
|---|---|---|---|
| Montana | Licensed Clinical Professional Counselor | | 60-semester-hour counseling-in-nature graduate degree from an accredited institution, including specific coursework and a 6-semester-hour advanced counseling practicum OR at least 45-semester-hour counseling-in-nature degree from an accredited institution, including a 6-semester-hour advanced counseling practicum; on board approval, the applicant must complete remaining hours to equal the total requirement of 60 semester hours |

| Clinical-Experience Requirements | Licensing Requirements[c] | License Renewal and Continuing Education | Independent Practice? | Health-Insurance Coverage[d] |
|---|---|---|---|---|
| 3,000 hours of supervised counseling experience under an LPC or licensed allied mental health professional, 1,500 hours of which must be postdegree; 1,000 of the 1,500 must be direct client contact | Applicant must have completed all degree and clinical-experience requirements, have passed the NCE or NCMHCE | License renewal annually; requires 20 contact hours | Yes—assessment, diagnosis, treatment planning, individual and group counseling | Mandated coverage |

*continued*

| State | Credentials[a] | Definition | Educational Requirements[b] |
|---|---|---|---|
| Nebraska | Licensed Independent Mental Health Practitioner; Licensed Mental Health Practitioner-Certified Professional Counselor *or* Licensed Professional Counselor; Licensed Mental Health Practitioner | LIMHP–CPC/LPC (new licensure tier as of June 1, 2007); a LMHP-CPC/LPC: available for LMHP who has a graduate degree from a CACREP-accredited program or a program with equivalent coursework; LMHP: a person who is qualified to engage in mental health practice or offers or renders mental health practice services | Master's degree or higher from an approved education program primarily therapeutic mental health in content and CACREP-accredited (or equivalent) from a regionally accredited institution and completion of a practicum or internship with at least 300 hours of direct client contact under the supervision of a qualified supervisor |

| Clinical-Experience Requirements | Licensing Requirements[c] | License Renewal and Continuing Education | Independent Practice? | Health-Insurance Coverage[d] |
|---|---|---|---|---|
| LIMHP: must have the LMHP credential and 2 years or 3,000 hours of post-master's experience in mental health practice accumulated in not more than 5 years under the supervision of an LIMHP, licensed psychologist, or licensed physician with mental health–treatment training, including 1,500 hours of experience with clients who have diagnoses of major mental illness; LMHP, LMHP–CPC/LPC: 3,000 hours of post-master's supervised experience in mental health practice accumulated during the 5 years immediately preceding the application for licensure, including 1,500 hours of direct client contact, with supervision under an LMHP, LIMHP, licensed psychologist, or licensed physician with mental health–treatment training | Applicant must have completed all degree and clinical-experience requirements, have passed the NCE or NCMHCE | License renewal every 2 years; requires 32 contact hours, 2 hours of continuing education in ethics | Yes, both LIMHPs and LMHP—assessment, treatment planning, individual and group counseling; LIMHPs may diagnose | |

*continued*

| State | Credentials[a] | Definition | Educational Requirements[b] |
| --- | --- | --- | --- |
| Nevada | Licensed Clinical Professional Counselor | | Master's degree or higher in mental health counseling or community counseling from a CACREP-accredited or equivalent program |
| New Hampshire | Licensed Clinical Mental Health Counselor | | Master's degree or higher in counseling or psychology from a regionally accredited institution with at least 2 academic years of full-time graduate study related to mental health counseling, 60 graduate semester hours, and coursework in nine content subjects |

| Clinical-Experience Requirements | Licensing Requirements[c] | License Renewal and Continuing Education | Independent Practice? | Health-Insurance Coverage[d] |
|---|---|---|---|---|
| 2 years or 3,000 hours of post-master's supervised counseling experience, including 1,500 hours of direct client contact and 100 hours of direct supervision | Applicant must have completed all degree and clinical-experience requirements, have passed the NCE or NCMHCE; NCE is accepted only if the applicant provides evidence of at least 3 years of work experience in mental health counseling; as of January 1, 2010, only the NCMHCE will be accepted | License renewal annually; no continuing-education requirement | Yes—assessment, diagnosis, treatment planning, individual and group counseling | |
| 2 years or 3,000 hours of paid post-master's supervised clinical work experience in a mental health setting to be completed in no more than 5 years, with at least 1,500 hours per year and 100 hours of face-to-face supervision provided by a licensed, board-approved mental health professional | Applicant must have completed all degree and clinical-experience requirements, have passed the NCMHCE and an essay examination | License renewal every 2 years; requires 40 contact hours, 6 hours of continuing education in ethics | Yes—assessment, diagnosis, treatment planning, individual and group counseling | Mandated coverage |

continued

| State | Credentials[a] | Definition | Educational Requirements[b] |
|---|---|---|---|
| New Jersey | Licensed Professional Counselor | | Master's degree in counseling from a regionally accredited institution with at least 60 graduate semester hours (45 of which must be distributed in eight of nine defined course-content subjects); an acceptable graduate degree is defined as one in which *"counseling"* or *"counselor"* appears in the title of the degree awarded or the institution offering the degree specifically states that the purpose of the graduate degree is to prepare students for the professional practice of counseling |

| Clinical-Experience Requirements | Licensing Requirements[c] | License Renewal and Continuing Education | Independent Practice? | Health-Insurance Coverage[d] |
|---|---|---|---|---|
| 3 years or 4,500 hours of full-time supervised counseling experience in a professional counseling setting, 1 year of which may be before master's degree is obtained; 30 graduate semester hours beyond the master's degree may be substituted for 1 year or 1,500 hours of experience; person must have at least 1 year of post-master's work experience | Applicant must be at least 18 years old, have completed all degree and clinical-experience requirements, have passed the NCE | License renewal every 2 years; requires 40 contact hours, 5 hours of continuing education in ethics and legal standards | Yes—assessment, diagnosis, treatment planning, individual and group counseling | |

continued

| State | Credentials[a] | Definition | Educational Requirements[b] |
|---|---|---|---|
| New Mexico | Licensed Professional Clinical Mental Health Counselor; Licensed Professional Mental Health Counselor; Licensed Mental Health Counselor | LPC: as of July 1, 2007, no longer issued; LMHC: a person who is pursuing a LPCC license but still needs to complete the supervised-experience requirements | LPCC: master's degree or higher in counseling or a counseling-related field (mental health, community counseling, agency counseling, psychology, clinical psychology, family studies, art therapy, or education) with at least 48 graduate hours from an accredited institution; LMHC: master's degree or higher in counseling or a counseling-related field with at least 48 graduate hours from an accredited institution and completion of 9 practicum hours |
| New York | Licensed Mental Health Counselor | | Master's degree or higher in counseling, including 48 semester hours and completion of specific coursework (requirement will increase to 60 hours on January 1, 2010), completion of 1-year supervised internship or practicum in mental health counseling (600 hours), and completion of coursework or training in the identification and reporting of child abuse |

| Clinical-Experience Requirements | Licensing Requirements[c] | License Renewal and Continuing Education | Independent Practice? | Health-Insurance Coverage[d] |
|---|---|---|---|---|
| LPCC: 2 years of postgraduate professional clinical counseling experience, including 3,000 hours of clinical client contact (1,000 of which may come from the graduate internship or practicum) and at least 100 hours of face-to-face supervision under an LPCC or licensed MFT, PAT, psychiatrist, clinical psychologist, or independent social worker | LPCC applicant must be at least 21 years old, have a master's or doctoral degree, have completed the required clinical experience, have passed the NCE or NCMHCE; LMHC (entry-level license) applicant must be at least 21 years old, have a master's degree, have completed 9 practicum hours, have passed the NCE | License renewal every 2 years; requires 40 contact hours, 6 hours of continuing education in ethics | Yes, LPCC—assessment, diagnosis, treatment planning, individual and group counseling | |
| 3,000 hours of post-master's supervised experience in providing mental health counseling | Applicant must be at least 21 years old; have completed all education, experience, and training requirements; have passed the NCMHCE | Registration renewal every 3 years; no continuing-education requirement | Yes—assessment, diagnosis, treatment planning, individual and group counseling | |

*continued*

| State | Credentials[a] | Definition | Educational Requirements[b] |
|---|---|---|---|
| North Carolina | Licensed Professional Counselor | | Master's degree or higher in counseling from a regionally accredited institution that includes 48 semester hours, coursework in eight content subjects, and a 300-hour practicum or internship OR master's degree or higher in a related field supplemented with equivalent coursework |

| Clinical-Experience Requirements | Licensing Requirements[c] | License Renewal and Continuing Education | Independent Practice? | Health-Insurance Coverage[d] |
|---|---|---|---|---|
| 2 years of post-master's counseling experience in a professional setting, including 2,000 hours of supervised professional practice (1,250 of which must be post-master's) and at least 100 hours of face-to-face supervision by a board-approved supervisor (with no more than 25 hours of group supervision) | Applicant must have a master's degree, have completed all clinical-experience requirements, have passed the NCE, NCMHCE, or CRCE | License renewal every 2 years; requires 40 contact hours, 3 hours of continuing education in ethics | Yes—assessment, diagnosis, treatment planning, individual and group counseling | |

*continued*

| State | Credentials[a] | Definition | Educational Requirements[b] |
|---|---|---|---|
| North Dakota | Licensed Professional Clinical Counselor; Licensed Professional Counselor; Licensed Associate Professional Counselor | LPC: full professional license after LAPC criteria are met and supervised experience has been completed; LAPC: a 2-year license that allows for completion of the supervised experience—requires 2-year plan of supervision and passing of the NCE | LPCC: master's degree or higher in counseling from an accredited institution, including 60 semester hours, core clinical coursework, and 800 hours of clinical training in a supervised practicum and internship; LPC/LAPC: master's degree or higher in counseling or a closely related field from an accredited institution, including 48 semester hours and specific core counseling coursework |

| Clinical-Experience Requirements | Licensing Requirements[c] | License Renewal and Continuing Education | Independent Practice? | Health-Insurance Coverage[d] |
|---|---|---|---|---|
| LPCC: must have the first-level LPC credential and 2 years or 3,000 hours of post-master's supervised clinical counseling experience in a clinical setting, including 100 hours of direct supervision by a board-approved supervisor, 60 of which must be individual face-to-face supervision; LPC: 400 hours of client counseling contact during the 2-year LAPC supervisory period, including 100 hours of direct supervision by a board-approved supervisor (of which 60 hours must be individual face-to-face supervision) | LPCC must have passed the NCMHCE, have completed a videotaped clinical counseling session of at least 30 minutes; LPC/LAPC must have passed the NCE | License renewal every 2 years; requires 30 contact hours for LPCs, 40 contact hours for LPCCs; LPCCs must also have 10 hours in clinical education | Yes, LPCCs and LPCs—assessment, diagnosis, treatment planning, individual and group counseling; LPC—allowed to practice independently in nonclinical settings | |

*continued*

| State | Credentials[a] | Definition | Educational Requirements[b] |
|---|---|---|---|
| Ohio | Licensed Professional Clinical Counselor; Licensed Professional Counselor | | Master's degree or higher in counseling (degrees in other disciplines, such as psychology, social work, and marriage and family therapy are not considered counseling degrees) from a CACREP- or CORE-accredited or equivalent program with 60 semester hours, 20 hours of which must be in clinical content subjects, and a 100-hour practicum and 600-hour internship |
| Oklahoma | Licensed Professional Counselor | | Master's degree or higher in counseling or a related mental health field with 60 graduate semester hours from a regionally accredited institution, including coursework in 10 subjects and a counseling practicum or internship of 300 hours |

| Clinical-Experience Requirements | Licensing Requirements[c] | License Renewal and Continuing Education | Independent Practice? | Health-Insurance Coverage[d] |
|---|---|---|---|---|
| LPCC: must have the first-level LPC credential and 2 years or 3,000 hours of post-master's clinical counseling experience under the supervision of an LPCC who has the supervision credential, including diagnosis of and treatment for mental and emotional disorders 50% of the time | LPCC must have passed the NCMHCE; LPC must have passed the NCE | License renewal every 2 years; requires 30 contact hours, 3 hours of continuing education in ethics and legal issues | Yes, LPCC and LPC—assessment, diagnosis, treatment planning, individual and group counseling | |
| 3 years or 3,000 hours of full-time postgraduate professional counseling experience supervised by an approved LPC supervisor; for each 1,000 hours, 350 hours must be direct face-to-face contact, and face-to-face supervision must be 45 minutes for every 20 hours of experience; 30 graduate semester hours beyond the master's degree may be substituted for every year of experience up to 2 years; person must have at least 1 year of supervised counseling experience | Applicant must be at least 21 years old; have successfully completed all related coursework, degree, and clinical-experience requirements; have passed the NCE and Oklahoma Legal and Ethical Responsibilities Examination | License renewal annually; requires 20 contact hours, 3 hours of continuing education in ethics | Yes—assessment, diagnosis, treatment planning, individual and group counseling | |

*continued*

| State | Credentials[a] | Definition | Educational Requirements[b] |
|---|---|---|---|
| Oregon | Licensed Professional Counselor | | Master's degree or higher in counseling with 48 semester hours in a CACREP- or CORE-accredited or equivalent program from a regionally accredited institution and a 600-hour internship or practicum |
| Pennsylvania | Licensed Professional Counselor | | Master's degree or higher in counseling or a closely related field from an accredited institution, including 60 semester hours and coursework in nine core subjects and a supervised practicum (100 hours) and internship (600 hours) |

| Clinical-Experience Requirements | Licensing Requirements[c] | License Renewal and Continuing Education | Independent Practice? | Health-Insurance Coverage[d] |
|---|---|---|---|---|
| 3 years of full-time supervised experience in counseling, including 2,400 hours of client contact and 120 hours of supervision (60 of which must be individual supervision) under an approved supervisor; 800 client contact hours may be obtained during the clinical portion of the qualifying degree program | Applicant must have completed all degree and clinical-experience requirements, have passed the NCE, NCMHCE, CRCE, or other examination approved by the state licensing board and the Oregon law and rules examination | License renewal annually; requires 40 contact hours every 2 years | Yes—assessment, diagnosis, treatment planning, individual and group counseling | |
| 3 years or 3,600 hours of supervised clinical experience under a qualified supervisor after completing 48 graduate-level credits; if person obtained doctorate in counseling: 2 years or 2,400 hours of supervised clinical experience, 1 year or 1,200 hours of which must be postdegree | Applicant must have completed all degree and clinical-experience requirements; have passed the NCE, CRCE, ATCB, CBMT, PEPK, AAODA, or EMAC | License renewal every 2 years; requires 30 contact hours, 3 hours of continuing education in ethics | Yes—assessment, diagnosis, treatment planning, individual and group counseling | |

continued

| State | Credentials[a] | Definition | Educational Requirements[b] |
|---|---|---|---|
| Puerto Rico | Licensed Professional Counselor | | Master's degree or higher in counseling from an institution accredited by the Council of Higher Education of Puerto Rico with specific coursework in 8 of 10 subjects |
| Rhode Island | Licensed Clinical Mental Health Counselor | | Master's degree or higher specializing in counseling or therapy from an institution accredited by the New England Association of Schools and Colleges or equivalent regional accrediting agency OR master's degree, certificate in advanced graduate studies, or doctoral degree in mental health counseling or allied field from a recognized educational institution AND, for both options, completion of 60 semester hours, coursework in eight core subjects, a supervised practicum (12 semester hours), and a 1-year supervised internship consisting of 20 hours per week in counseling |

| Clinical-Experience Requirements | Licensing Requirements[c] | License Renewal and Continuing Education | Independent Practice? | Health-Insurance Coverage[d] |
|---|---|---|---|---|
| At least 500 hours of post-master's practice supervised by a certified mentor (licensed LPC certified by the board to supervise) | Applicant must have passed the NCE | License renewal every 3 years; requires 45 contact hours | Yes | |
| 2 years or 2,000 hours of post-master's direct client contact offering clinical counseling or therapy services with emphasis on mental health counseling, including 100 hours of supervised case work under a board-approved supervisor over the 2-year period | Applicant must have completed all degree and clinical-experience requirements, have passed the NCMHCE | License renewal every 2 years; requires 40 contact hours | Yes—assessment, diagnosis, treatment planning, individual and group counseling | Mandated coverage |

*continued*

| State | Credentials[a] | Definition | Educational Requirements[b] |
|---|---|---|---|
| South Carolina | Licensed Professional Counselor; Professional Counselor Intern | LPC/I: a person who has met the education and examination requirements but not the requirement of 2 years of supervised experience | Master's degree or higher in professional counseling or related discipline from a regionally accredited institution, including at least 48 semester hours, coursework in 10 content subjects, and a 150-hour supervised counseling practicum |

| Clinical-Experience Requirements | Licensing Requirements[c] | License Renewal and Continuing Education | Independent Practice? | Health-Insurance Coverage[d] |
| --- | --- | --- | --- | --- |
| Must have the first-level LPC/I credential and 2 years or 1,500 hours of full-time post-master's supervised clinical experience in the practice of professional counseling involving direct counseling with individuals, couples, families, or groups, including at least 150 hours of clinical supervision by a board-approved LPC supervisor (100 hours must be individual supervision) | Applicant must be credentialed as an LPC/I, have passed the NCE or NCMHCE | License renewal every 2 years; requires 40 contact hours | Yes—assessment, diagnosis, treatment planning, individual and group counseling | |

continued

| State | Credentials[a] | Definition | Educational Requirements[b] |
|---|---|---|---|
| South Dakota | Licensed Professional Counselor-Mental Health; Licensed Professional Counselor | | Master's degree or higher with an emphasis in mental health counseling from a CACREP-accredited or equivalent program that includes specific coursework and a supervised practicum (100 hours) and internship (600 hours); LPC: 48 semester hours; LPC-MH: 60 semester hours or completion of all required coursework |

| Clinical-Experience Requirements | Licensing Requirements[c] | License Renewal and Continuing Education | Independent Practice? | Health-Insurance Coverage[d] |
|---|---|---|---|---|
| LPC-MH: must have the first-level LPC credential and 2 years or 2,000 hours of post-master's direct client contact in a clinical setting, including 100 hours of face-to-face supervision; 1,000 hours of post-master's direct client contact and 50 hours of face-to-face supervision earned under the LPC credential may be counted toward these requirements; LPC: 2,000 hours of full-time post-master's counseling experience, including 800 hours of direct client contact and 100 hours of face-to-face supervision | LPC-MH must have passed the NCMHCE; LPC must have passed the NCE | License renewal annually; requires 40 contact hours every 2 years | Yes, LPC and LPC-MH—assessment, diagnosis, treatment planning, individual and group counseling | Mandated coverage, mandated offering |

continued

| State | Credentials[a] | Definition | Educational Requirements[b] |
|---|---|---|---|
| Tennessee | Licensed Professional Counselor-Mental Health Service Provider; Licensed Professional Counselor | | LPC/MHSP: in addition to or as part of the graduate degree, completion of 9 graduate semester hours of coursework related to diagnosis, appraisal, and assessment of and treatment for mental disorders; LPC: 60 graduate semester hours in professional counseling or a related field from an institution accredited by the Southern Association of Colleges and Schools, CACREP, or a comparable accrediting body, including completion of a master's degree in professional counseling and a supervised 500-hour practicum or internship (300 hours of which must be completed in a clinical setting) |

| Clinical-Experience Requirements | Licensing Requirements[c] | License Renewal and Continuing Education | Independent Practice? | Health-Insurance Coverage[d] |
|---|---|---|---|---|
| 2 years of post-master's professional experience consisting of 3,000 hours of direct clinical experience (at least 10 hours per week) and 50 hours of supervision per week | Applicant must be at least 18 years old, have completed all educational and clinical-experience requirements; LPC/MHSP must have passed the NCE, NCMHCE, and Tennessee Jurisprudence Examination for Professional Counselors; LPC must have passed the NCE and Tennessee Jurisprudence Examination for Professional Counselors | License renewal every 2 years; requires 20 contact hours (10 per year), 3 hours of continuing education per year in ethics or Tennessee code, rules, or regulations | Yes, LPC/MHSP and LPC—assessment, diagnosis, treatment planning, individual and group counseling | |

continued

| State | Credentials[a] | Definition | Educational Requirements[b] |
| --- | --- | --- | --- |
| Texas | Licensed Professional Counselor | | Master's degree or higher in professional counseling or related field (including psychology, psychiatry, social work, marriage and family therapy, and guidance and counseling) consisting of 48 graduate semester hours from an accredited institution, including completion of specific coursework and a 300-hour supervised practicum with at least 100 hours of direct client contact |
| Utah | Licensed Professional Counselor | | Master's degree or higher in mental health counseling from a CACREP-accredited program, including at least 60 graduate semester hours in specific coursework, 3 semester hours of a practicum, and 6 semester hours of an internship |

| Clinical-Experience Requirements | Licensing Requirements[c] | License Renewal and Continuing Education | Independent Practice? | Health-Insurance Coverage[d] |
|---|---|---|---|---|
| 3 years or 3,000 hours of post-master's supervised experience under a board-approved LPC, including 1,500 hours of direct client contact | Applicant must have a graduate degree from an approved program, have completed all clinical-experience requirements, have passed the NCE and Texas Jurisprudence Examination | License renewal every 2 years; requires 24 contact hours (12 per year), 3 hours of continuing education in ethics every 2 years | Yes—assessment, diagnosis, treatment planning, individual and group counseling | Mandated coverage |
| 2 years or 4,000 hours of post-master's supervised professional counseling experience, 1,000 of which must be supervised experience in mental health therapy, including 100 hours of face-to-face supervision by a licensed mental health therapist | Applicant must have completed all degree-program, coursework, and clinical-experience requirements; have passed the NCE, NCMHCE, and the Utah Professional Counselor Law, Rules and Ethics Examination | License renewal every 2 years; requires 40 contact hours | Yes—assessment, diagnosis, treatment planning, individual and group counseling | Mandated coverage |

*continued*

| State | Credentials[a] | Definition | Educational Requirements[b] |
| --- | --- | --- | --- |
| Vermont | Licensed Clinical Mental Health Counselor | | Master's degree or higher in counseling from an accredited institution with a minimum of 60 semester hours and 1,000 hours of a supervised practicum, internship, or field experience in a clinical mental health setting |
| Virginia | Licensed Professional Counselor | | Master's degree or higher in counseling or related field, including 60 semester hours from a program that reflects the CACREP or CORE curriculum, and completion of a supervised internship of at least 600 hours |

| Clinical-Experience Requirements | Licensing Requirements[c] | License Renewal and Continuing Education | Independent Practice? | Health-Insurance Coverage[d] |
|---|---|---|---|---|
| 2 years or 3,000 hours of post-master's experience in clinical mental health counseling, including 2,000 hours of direct client contact and 100 hours of face-to-face supervision under a board-approved licensed mental health professional | Applicant must have received a graduate degree, completed the minimum number of hours of clinical experience, and passed the NCE and NCMHCE | Licensure renewal every 2 years; requires 40 contact hours and 4 hours continuing education in ethics | Yes—assessment, diagnosis, treatment planning, and individual/group counseling | Mandated offering |
| 4,000 hours of postgraduate supervised counseling experience, including 2,000 hours of direct client contact and 200 hours of face-to-face supervision (of which 100 hours must be individual supervision with an LPC and 100 can be group supervision); graduate-level internship hours may count toward the 4,000 hours, depending on the program | Applicant must have completed all degree-program, coursework, and clinical-experience requirements; have passed the NCMHCE | License renewal annually; requires 20 contact hours, 2 hours of continuing education in ethics | Yes—assessment, diagnosis, treatment planning, individual and group counseling | Mandated coverage |

continued

| State | Credentials[a] | Definition | Educational Requirements[b] |
|---|---|---|---|
| Washington | Licensed Mental Health Counselor | | Master's degree or higher in mental health counseling or related field from a regionally accredited institution, including a supervised counseling practicum or internship and 4 hours of HIV/AIDS education and training |
| West Virginia | Licensed Professional Counselor | | Master's degree or higher (acceptable degrees: specialization in community agency counseling, mental health counseling, pastoral counseling, rehabilitation counseling, school counseling, substance-abuse or addiction counseling, or similar degrees that include *"counseling"* deemed closely related by the board) from a CACREP- or CORE-accredited program or comparable accrediting body with 60 semester hours and a practicum and internship |

| Clinical-Experience Requirements | Licensing Requirements[c] | License Renewal and Continuing Education | Independent Practice? | Health-Insurance Coverage[d] |
|---|---|---|---|---|
| 3 years of full-time counseling or 3,000 hours of postgraduate supervised mental health counseling in an approved setting, including 1,200 hours of direct counseling with individuals, couples, groups, or families and 100 hours of immediate supervision by a board-approved supervisor | Applicant must have a graduate degree, have completed all clinical-experience requirements, have passed the NCE or NCMHCE | License renewal annually; requires 36 contact hours every 2 years, 6 hours of continuing education in ethics and law | Yes—assessment, diagnosis, treatment planning, individual and group counseling | Mandated coverage |
| 2 years or 3,000 hours of post-master's supervised professional counseling experience under a board-approved professional, of which at least 50% is in the direct provision of counseling services to clients and which includes at least 1 hour of direct individual supervision for every 20 hours of practice | Applicant must have a graduate degree, have completed all clinical-experience requirements, have passed the NCE or CRCE | License renewal every 2 years; requires 40 contact hours, 3 hours of continuing education in ethics | Yes—assessment, diagnosis, treatment planning, individual and group counseling | |

continued

| State | Credentials[a] | Definition | Educational Requirements[b] |
| --- | --- | --- | --- |
| Wisconsin | Licensed Professional Counselor | | Master's degree or higher in professional counseling or equivalent program from a regionally accredited institution with at least 42 semester hours, including 3 semester hours of counseling theories and 3 semester hours of supervised counseling |
| Wyoming | Licensed Professional Counselor | | Master's degree or higher in counseling with at least 48 semester hours from a CACREP- or CORE-accredited program or regionally accredited institution |

NOTE: This summary should not be relied upon as a definitive source of information on license requirements—state license boards should always be consulted for current and complete requirements.

[a]CPC = certified professional counselor, LAC = licensed associate counselor, LAPC = licensed associate professional counselor, LCMHC = licensed clinical mental health counselor, LCPC = licensed clinical professional counselor, LIMHP = licensed independent mental health practitioner, LMHC = licensed mental health counselor, LMHP = licensed mental health practitioner, LPC = licensed professional counselor,

| Clinical-Experience Requirements | Licensing Requirements[c] | License Renewal and Continuing Education | Independent Practice? | Health-Insurance Coverage[d] |
|---|---|---|---|---|
| 2 years or 3,000 hours of post-master's supervised professional counseling practice, including 1,000 hours of face-to-face client contact and 1 hour of face-to-face supervision per week by a board-approved mental health professional | Applicant must have a master's or doctoral degree, have completed all clinical-experience requirements, have passed the NCE, NCMHCE, CRCE, or equivalent examination and the Wisconsin jurisprudence examination | License renewal every 2 years; requires 30 contact hours | Yes—assessment, diagnosis, treatment planning, individual and group counseling | |
| 3,000 hours of supervised clinical experience (1,500 of which must be post-master's), including 100 hours of face-to-face supervision by a licensed mental health professional | Applicant must be 18 years old, have a master's or doctoral degree, have completed all clinical-experience requirements, have passed the NCE | License renewal every 2 years; requires 45 contact hours | Yes—assessment, diagnosis, treatment planning, individual and group counseling | Mandated coverage |

LPCC = licensed professional clinical counselor, LPC/I = licensed professional counselor intern, LPC-MH = licensed professional counselor of mental health, LPCMHC = licensed professional clinical mental health counselor, LPC/MHSP = licensed professional counselor/mental health service provider, LPMHC = licensed professional mental health counselor

[b]CACREP = Council for Accreditation of Counseling and Related Educational Programs (organizational affiliate of American Counseling Association), CCMHC = certified clinical mental health counselor, CHEA = Council for Higher Education Accreditation,

*continued*

CORE = Council on Rehabilitation Education, *DSM* = *Diagnostic and Statistical Manual of Mental Disorders*, NBCC = National Board for Certified Counselors.
[c]AAODA = Advanced Alcohol and Other Drug Abuse Counselor (examination administered by the International Certification and Reciprocity Consortium/Alcohol and Other Drug Abuse, Inc.), ATCB = Art Therapy Credentials Board, CBMT = Certification Board for Music Therapists, CRCE = Certified Rehabilitation Counselor Examination, EMAC = Examination for Master Addictions Counselors (administered by National Board for Certified Counselors), NCE = National Counselor Examination (administered by National Board for Certified Counselors), NCMHCE = National Clinical Mental Health Counselor Examination (administered by National Board for Certified Counselors), PEPK = Practice Examination of Psychological Knowledge (administered by Northamerican Association of Masters in Psychology).
[d]*Mandated coverage* (or freedom of choice) refers to laws that mandate that specific provider groups be reimbursed for their services when the services are covered by a health plan. *Mandated offering* refers to laws that require insurers to offer the services of a provider when the services are covered by a health plan. *Any willing provider* refers to laws that require managed-care organizations to contract with any qualified provider who agrees to meet the contractual terms and conditions of the plan.

# Appendix H

# Biographic Sketches of Committee Members, Consultant, and Staff

**George J. Isham, MD, MS** (*Chair*), is chief health officer and plan medical director of HealthPartners, the largest consumer-governed, nonprofit health-care organization in the nation. He is past cochair and current member of the National Committee for Quality Assurance Committee on Performance Measurement, which oversees quality-measurement standards. Dr. Isham is also a member of the National Priority Partners effort convened by the National Quality Forum and chairs the population-health work group of the effort. Before his present position, he was medical director of MedCenters Health Plan in Minneapolis and was executive director of University Health Care, an organization affiliated with the University of Wisconsin–Madison. His practice experience includes service as a medical officer in the US Navy. He was chair of the Institute of Medicine (IOM) committee that produced the report *Priority Areas for National Action: Transforming Health Care Quality* and a member of the Subcommittee on Performance Measurement of IOM's Committee on Redesigning Health Insurance Performance Measures, Payment, and Performance Improvement Programs. He is currently chair of IOM's Roundtable on Health Literacy. Dr. Isham received his medical degree from the University of Illinois and served his internship and residency in internal medicine at the University of Wisconsin Hospital and Clinics in Madison. He also holds an MS in preventive medicine and administrative medicine from the University of Wisconsin–Madison. Dr. Isham is a National Associate of the Institute of Medicine.

**Kathryn Karusaitis Basham, PhD, LICSW,** is professor in the Smith College School for Social Work, Co-Director of the doctoral program, and editor of *Smith College Studies in Social Work*. Her fields of research, publication, and teaching interest include clinical practice models with survivors of childhood trauma and combat trauma, couple- and family-therapy practice after deployment, cross-cultural practice, pedagogy, diversity and antiracism practice, ethics, and professional identity development. Recent publications and teaching consultations have focused on couple- and family-therapy approaches with service members and their families at the Walter Reed Army Medical Center (Washington, DC) and several Veterans Administration Medical Centers throughout the country and with military and civilian clinicians working with Canadian Forces. Dr. Basham has previously served as a committee member in Institute of Medicine studies that resulted in the reports *Posttraumatic Stress Disorder: Diagnosis and Assessment* (2006) and *Gulf War and Health, Volume 6: Physiologic, Psychologic, and Psychosocial Effects of Deployment-Related Stress* (2008). She was coauthor of a text titled *Transforming the Legacy: Couple Therapy with Survivors of Childhood Trauma* (2004). Dr. Basham maintains a private practice in clinical social work, specializing in couple, family, and individual psychotherapy and consultation services. In collaboration with a colleague at Smith College, she is engaged in a pilot research project that explores the effectiveness of a couple-therapy practice model for traumatized couples in which one partner is a veteran of Operation Iraqi Freedom and had a diagnosis of posttraumatic stress disorder. In 2007, she was inducted into the National Academies of Practice as a distinguished practitioner and has worked actively on issues pertaining to graduate-level education for social workers and licensure. Dr. Basham earned her MSW from the University of California, Berkeley, and her PhD from Smith College.

**Alisa B. Busch, MD, MS,** is assistant professor of psychiatry and of health-care policy at Harvard Medical School. She is also director of integration of clinical measurement and health services research at McLean Hospital. Dr. Busch has over 10 years of experience in treating patients who have psychiatric illness, most recently as attending psychiatrist at McLean's Alcohol and Drug Abuse Partial Hospital Program. Dr. Busch's primary research interests are in measuring the quality of mental health care and understanding how systemwide policy and financing arrangements affect the quality of mental health treatment. She has examined quality of care in the public and private sectors for psychiatric illnesses, including depression, bipolar disorder, schizophrenia, and co-occurring substance-use disorders. In 2004, she was awarded the McLean Hospital Alfred Pope Award for Young Investigators for her research on the effect of a Medicaid managed behavioral health carveout on quality of care for schizophrenia. Dr. Busch is a current recipient of a Career Development Award from the National Institute of Mental Health to conduct research on quality of care for bipolar disorder. She is also a network member in the MacArthur Foundation Research Network on Mandated Community Treatment. Dr. Busch received a BA in English from New York University, her MD from the Johns Hopkins University School of Medicine, and her MS in health policy and management from the Harvard School of Public Health.

**N. Emmanuel (Manoli) G. Cassimatis, MD,** is president and chief executive officer of the Educational Commission for Foreign Medical Graduates (ECFMG) and chair of the Foundation for Advancement of International Medical Education and Research, ECFMG's nonprofit foundation. He was formerly vice president for affiliations and international affairs at the Uniformed Services University of the Health Sciences (USUHS), associate dean for clinical affairs and professor of psychiatry at the University's F. Edward Hébert School of Medicine. He served in the US Army for 26 years and retired with the rank of colonel. Earlier in his career, he practiced at the Walter Reed Army Medical Center, serving as assistant chief of the Inpatient Psychiatry Service, director of Psychiatric Education and Training, and chief of the Outpatient Psychiatry Service. Later assignments included a tour as deputy commander for clinical services at the Army's Frankfurt Regional Medical Center and positions in the Office of the Army Surgeon General as psychiatry consultant; chief of the Graduate Medical Education Branch, and Chief of the Medical Education Division. Dr. Cassimatis served on the Accreditation Council for Graduate Medical Education (ACGME) Institutional Review Committee from 2001 through 2004 and on the ACGME Board of Directors from 1999 to 2006, the last 2 years as chair. From 1995 through 1997, he was a delegate to the American Medical Association (AMA) House of Delegates from the Association of Military Surgeons of the United States (AMSUS) and served as a member and chair of the AMA Council on Medical Education, the AMA Specialty and Service Society Governing Council, the AMA Section Council on

Federal and Military Medicine, and the American Board of Medical Specialties–AMA Liaison Committee on Specialty Boards. In addition to his duties at USUHS, Dr. Cassimatis serves on the Executive Committee of the National Disaster Life Support Education Consortium and as president of the Hellenic American Psychiatric Association. Dr. Cassimatis received his BA from the University of Chicago, his MD from Harvard Medical School, and his psychoanalytic training at the Washington Psychoanalytic Institute. He is a Life Fellow of AMSUS, a member of the Academy of Medicine of Washington, DC, a fellow of the American Academy of Psychoanalysis and Dynamic Psychiatry, and a Distinguished Life Fellow of the American Psychiatric Association.

**John H. Moxley III, MD,** is an independent consultant and is the retired managing director of the North American Health Care Division of Korn/Ferry International. His expertise includes training, costs, and manpower issues; federal-agency administration; and military medical issues. He has held a number of senior positions in academe, government, and industry, including being dean of the medical schools of the University of Maryland and the University of California, San Diego; Assistant Secretary of Defense for Health Affairs; and senior vice president of the hospital management firm American Medical International. Dr. Moxley has served on numerous scientific boards and advisory committees, including the American Hospital Association Board of Trustees; the Scientific Board of the California Medical Association, as chairman; the Council on Scientific Affairs of the American Medical Association; the National Fund for Medical Education; and the Henry M. Jackson Foundation for the Advancement of Military Medicine. He was chair of the National Research Council Committee on Strategies to Protect the Health of Deployed US Forces and served on the Research Council's Board on Army Science and Technology and Naval Studies Board. Dr. Moxley earned his MD from the University of Colorado; he is board-certified in internal medicine and is a fellow of the American College of Physicians. He is a member of the Institute of Medicine.

**Harold A. Pincus, MD,** is professor and vice chair of the Department of Psychiatry and associate director of the Irving Institute for Clinical and Translational Research at Columbia University. He is also director of quality and outcomes research at New York–Presbyterian Hospital and serves as a senior scientist at the RAND Corporation. Dr. Pincus is the director of the Robert Wood Johnson Foundation's Depression in Primary Care: Linking Clinical and Systems Strategies program. He previously served as deputy medical director of the American Psychiatric Association and was the founding director of its Office of Research, executive director of the American Psychiatric Institute for Research and Education, cochair of the work group to update the text of the *Diagnostic and Statistical Manual, Fourth Edition*, and special assistant to the director of the National Institute of Mental Health. He has published widely in health-services research, science policy, and the diagnosis and classification of and treatment for mental disorders, and he has been appointed to the editorial boards of 10 major scientific journals. Dr. Pincus is the principal investigator of the congressionally mandated Program Evaluation of Mental Health Services in the Veterans Health Administration of the Department of Veterans Affairs. He graduated from the University of Pennsylvania and received his MD from Albert Einstein College of Medicine in New York. Dr. Pincus maintains a small private practice specializing in major affective disorders and has spent one evening a week for 22 years at a public mental health clinic caring for patients who have severe mental illness.

**Theodore P. Remley, Jr., JD, PhD, LPC,** is professor and Batten Endowed Chair in the Counseling Graduate Program at Old Dominion University in Virginia, where he is chair of the Department of Counseling and Human Services. Before joining the faculty at Old Dominion University, Dr. Remley led counseling doctoral programs at the University of New Orleans and Mississippi State University and was executive director of the American Counseling Association (ACA) from 1990 to 1994. He has served as a school counselor and a college counselor and has had a private practice in both counseling and law. He has expertise in licensure, certification, private practice, and employment and public recognition of counselors, and he is the first author of the counselor-education text *Ethical, Legal, and Professional Issues in Counseling*. Dr. Remley holds a doctorate in counselor education from the University of Florida and a law degree from Catholic University in Washington, DC. He served in the US Army Reserve and the Virginia Army National Guard, earning the rank of captain. He is a licensed professional counselor in Virginia, Louisiana, and Mississippi and is a member of the bar in Virginia and Florida. A nationally certified counselor, he has chaired the counselor-licensure boards in Virginia and Mississippi and served as a member of the Louisiana and District of Columbia boards. Dr. Remley was named an ACA fellow in 2008 for his service and scholarship contributions to the counseling profession, one of the highest awards given by ACA.

**Phyllis W. Sharps, PhD, RN, CNE, FAAN,** is professor and chair of the Department of Community Public Health at the Johns Hopkins University School of Nursing and the director of three health and wellness centers operated by the school. Dr. Sharps conducts community-based participatory research and has a current study funded by the National Institutes of Health to examine community-health nurse interventions for abused pregnant women aimed at reducing violent victimization and improving maternal physical, mental, and other health outcomes. The overarching focus of her work is on the effects of intimate-partner violence on the physical and emotional health of pregnant women, infants, and very young children. Research activities have included investigations of mental health, depression, and other factors that affect the health of military pregnant women. Dr. Sharps applies her clinical research findings to improving women's health through her activities as a member of the Advisory Board for the International Association of Chiefs of Police and as a trainer and consultant for the Family Violence Prevention Fund and National Institute of Justice. She is consulted frequently about cultural competence in research with African American women and communities. She earned her PhD from the University of Maryland School of Nursing. Dr. Sharps served in the US Army (active duty and Reserves in the Nurse Corps) for 30 years, retiring with the rank of colonel.

**Roy A. Swift, PhD, FAOTA,** is senior director of personnel credentialing accreditation programs for the American National Standards Institute. Before his current position, he was a consultant to educational, certification, licensure, and health-care organizations. From 1993 to 1998, he was executive director of the National Board for Certification in Occupational Therapy. That appointment followed a career in the US Army Medical Department. In his last position, he was chief of the Army Medical Specialist Corps with policy responsibility for Army occupational therapists, physical therapists, dietitians, and physician assistants throughout the world. Dr. Swift serves on the Board of Directors of CGFNS International and as a member of the Board of Directors Standing Hearing Panel of the American Psychological Association. He has served on the Board of Directors of the Council on Licensure, Enforcement and Regulation and the National Organization for Competency Assurance. He has also served on national committees with the American Occupational Therapy Association, including being chair of the accreditation committee for academic programs, and chaired the Assembly of Review Committee Chairmen of the former Council on Allied Health Education and Accreditation of the American Medical Association. From July 2003 to October 2006, Dr. Swift served on the Secretary of Veterans Affairs' Professional Certification and Licensure Advisory Committee. He received a BS in occupational therapy from the University of Kansas, an MS from the University of Southern California, and a PhD in continuing and vocational education from the University of Wisconsin–Madison. He served in the US Army for 28 years, retiring with the rank of colonel.

**Vilia M. Tarvydas, PhD, CRC, LMHC,** is professor and clinical coordinator for the Graduate Programs in Rehabilitation in the Department of Counseling, Rehabilitation, and Student Development of the University of Iowa College of Education. Dr. Tarvydas is a certified rehabilitation counselor and a licensed mental health counselor with more than 33 years of experience as a rehabilitation counselor educator and practicing rehabilitation professional. Her scholarly works and professional presentations have concentrated on ethics and ethical decision making, professional standards, and rehabilitation after traumatic brain injury. The third edition of her textbook, *Counseling Ethics and Decision Making,* was published in 2007. In 2008, she received two prominent awards for her career contributions: the James F. Garrett Distinguished Career Research Award from the American Rehabilitation Counseling Association (ARCA) and the Distinguished Career in Rehabilitation Education Award from the National Council on Rehabilitation Education (NCRE). She has been prominent in leadership of the major professional organizations in counseling and rehabilitation counseling, serving on the Board of Directors of the National Rehabilitation Counseling Association, as vice chair of the Commission on Rehabilitation Counselor Certification, and as president of ARCA and NCRE. She is president of the American Association of State Counseling Boards and immediate past chair of the Iowa Board of Behavior Examiners and chair of its Disciplinary Committee. She has served as a member of the American Counseling Association's Ethics Committee and the Judicial Council of the American Occupational Therapy Association. Recently, Dr. Tarvydas developed the Institute on

Disability and Rehabilitation Ethics in the University of Iowa College of Education. Dr. Tarvydas received her MA in educational rehabilitation counseling and her PhD in rehabilitation psychology from the University of Wisconsin–Madison.

### *Consultant to the Committee*

**Rhonda J. Robinson Beale, MD,** is the chief medical officer for OptumHealth Behavioral Solutions, a health-maintenance organization. Earlier, she served as the chief medical officer for PacifiCare Behavioral Health, senior vice president and chief medical officer for CIGNA Behavioral Health, national medical director for Blue Cross Blue Shield, executive medical director of medical and care management clinical programs for Blue Cross Blue Shield of Michigan, and senior medical director for behavioral medicine for Health Alliance Plan. Dr. Robinson Beale has over 20 years of behavioral health and quality-management experience. She is a member of the Institute of Medicine (IOM) Board on Health Care Services and has served on the IOM Board on Neuroscience and Behavioral Health. As a member of several IOM committees, Dr. Robinson Beale has contributed to important national studies, including *Crossing the Quality Chasm* and *Managing Managed Care: Quality Improvement in Behavioral Health.* In addition, she has served on the National Quality Forum Board of Directors as cochair of the Steering Committee for Evidence-Based Practices to Treat Substance Use Disorders project. She serves on the Board of Directors of the Association for Behavioral Health and Wellness. Dr. Robinson Beale received her medical degree from the Wayne State University School of Medicine and her psychiatric training at the Detroit Psychiatric Institute. She is certified in psychiatry by the American Board of Psychiatry and Neurology. Dr. Robinson Beale is a National Associate of IOM.

### *Institute of Medicine Staff and Other Contributors*

**David A. Butler, PhD,** is senior program officer in the Institute of Medicine (IOM) Board on the Health of Select Populations. He received his BS and MS in engineering from the University of Rochester and his PhD in public-policy analysis from Carnegie Mellon University. Before joining IOM, Dr. Butler served as an analyst for the US Congress Office of Technology Assessment and was Research Associate in the Department of Environmental Health of the Harvard School of Public Health. He has directed several IOM studies on military-health topics, including ones that produced *PTSD Compensation and Military Service, Veterans and Agent Orange: Update 1998* and *Update 2000, Disposition of the Air Force Health Study*, and the series *Characterizing the Exposure of Veterans to Agent Orange and Other Herbicides Used in Vietnam: Scientific Considerations Regarding a Request for Proposals for Research*. Dr. Butler was also a coeditor of *Systems Engineering to Improve Traumatic Brain Injury Care in the Military Health System: Workshop Summary*.

**Jessica L. Buono, MPH,** is a fellow at Merck & Co., Inc., conducting pharmacoeconomics and outcomes research. Earlier, she worked as research associate with the Board on the Health of Select Populations of the Institute of Medicine. She has also held positions as a research associate in the Policy and Global Affairs division of the National Academies and as a Christine Mirzayan Science and Technology Policy Fellow for the National Academy of Engineering Program Office and the Committee on Women in Science, Engineering, and Medicine. Ms. Buono received her BS in behavioral neuroscience from Lehigh University and her MPH in epidemiology from the George Washington University.

**Sarah Gaillot, MPhil,** was a Christine Mirzayan Science and Technology Policy Fellow for the Institute of Medicine Board on the Health of Select Populations. She is completing a PhD in policy analysis at the Pardee RAND Graduate School (PRGS), where her research focuses on disparities in the use of trauma and mental health service. She also serves as an assistant policy analyst at RAND, focusing on military health policy. Before joining PRGS and RAND, Ms. Gaillot taught English in South Korea on a Fulbright teaching grant. She received a BS in human development–family studies and psychology from Pennsylvania State University and spent semesters at the University of Ghana and the National University of Singapore.

**Andrew Bradley, BS,** graduated from the University of Virginia (UVa), where he majored in biomedical engineering, in 2008. Through the UVa School of Engineering's Policy Internship Program, he interned in 2007 at the Institute of Medicine for the Board on Military and Veterans Health. He is a pursuing his medical studies at the University of Michigan.

**Frederick (Rick) Erdtmann, MD, MPH,** is director of the Board on the Health of Select Populations and of the Medical Follow-up Agency of the Institute of Medicine. He earned his MD from Temple University School of Medicine, and he holds an MPH from the University of California, Berkeley. He completed a residency program in general preventive medicine at Walter Reed Army Institute of Research in 1975 and is board certified in that specialty. Dr. Erdtmann's assignments with the Army Medical Department included being chief of preventive-medicine services at Fitzsimons Army Medical Center, at Frankfurt Army Medical Center in Germany, and at Madigan Army Medical Center. He also served as division surgeon for the Second Infantry Division in Tongduchon, Korea. He later served as Deputy Chief of Staff for Clinical Operations in the Department of Defense's TRICARE Region 1 before assuming hospital command at Walter Reed Army Medical Center in March 1998. After that, he was assigned to the Office of the Surgeon General as the Deputy Assistant Surgeon General for Force Development. In 2001, after 30 years of commissioned military service, Dr. Erdtmann joined the National Academies and assumed his present responsibilities.

**Pamela Ramey-McCray, BA,** joined the National Academies in 1993 as a senior project assistant for the Medical Follow-up Agency and has been the administrative assistant for the Institute of Medicine Board on the Health of Selection Populations since 1996. Ms. Ramey-McCray graduated from Trinity College, where she majored in human relations, in 2004. She is a member of Psi Chi, the International Honor Society in Psychology.